SPEAKING TO POWER
Advocacy for health and social care

David Donnison

D1460628

P

First published in Great Britain in 2009 by

Policy Press   North America office:
University of Bristol   Policy Press
1-9 Old Park Hill   c/o The University of Chicago Press
Bristol   1427 East 60th Street
BS2 8BB   Chicago, IL 60637, USA
UK   t: +1 773 702 7700
t: +44 (0)117 954 5940   f: +1 773-702-9756
pp-info@bristol.ac.uk   sales@press.uchicago.edu
www.policypress.co.uk   www.press.uchicago.edu

© Policy Press 2009

British Library Cataloguing in Publication Data
A catalogue record for this book is available from the British Library.

Library of Congress Cataloging-in-Publication Data
A catalog record for this book has been requested.

ISBN 978 1 84742 037 4 paperback
ISBN 978 1 84742 038 1 hardcover

Cover design by Qube Design Associates, Bristol
Printed and bound in Great Britain by Marston Book Services, Oxford

This book is dedicated to David Brandon (1941–2001), mental health services user and practitioner, scholar, teacher and advocate.

Contents

Why and how we wrote this book

This book was inspired by the Scottish service that provides advocacy to help people with mental health or learning difficulties. Advocacy for these and other groups began earlier in other countries of the UK, but nowhere else is there the free and independent nationwide service that is to be found in Scotland. When I first got involved, staff of the agency I joined asked where they could find opportunities for further training and professional development. Few were available. No surprise there: the academy always lags about a decade behind new developments in the field because their teachers need a shelf of books to read before they can offer a course, and it takes time to do the research and writing that creates this literature.

So we said, "Let's write our own book". We worked on it in small meetings of advocates held in various parts of the territory our agency serves: a territory including old industrial towns, comfortable suburbs, and smaller communities scattered among mountains, lochs and islands; a territory with a population of nearly 200,000 people and a coastline longer than the coast of France. Very Scottish.

Central among the readers for whom we have written the book are people working as advocates or preparing to do so in Scotland or elsewhere. We hope our book will also be helpful to users of the mental health services, to those who care for them, the professionals who try to help them, and anyone interested in the broader development of the health and social services.

Our advocates brought anonymous but real cases to discuss with their colleagues at our meetings. To these we added a few others from colleagues working elsewhere in the same cause. I brought draft chapters, which were freely criticised and, in 18 months we created this book. We also sought the help of others who are expert in this field and asked some of them to comment on the whole draft or on particular chapters of it.

We could not have written the book without the help of our clients. Some of them wrote their own stories for us. Others gave their advocates permission to do this for them. We are grateful to them all. To protect confidentiality we have disguised these stories with small changes that preserve their essential truths. We have not mentioned the names of clients or places; and their advocates' names are only acknowledged in this preface.

People tend to seek the help of an advocate when things go wrong for them. They may feel they are the victims of incompetence, injustice or worse; and they may be right. Thus the glimpses we give of the work of public services are often unflattering and may be unfair. There is another side to every story, but our promise of confidentiality for our clients precluded us from asking about that. So we invited spokesmen of the main services involved to read and comment on the relevant chapters. We are grateful for their help.

At the end of the day, someone has to do most of the writing for a book of this kind. Someone has to edit other people's contributions, find a publisher, correct the proofs and prepare an index. And take the blame for any errors left in the book. That's why my name appears on the cover.

Working with a team of people who are engaged in a cause of this kind to which they are deeply committed has been a marvellous experience for me. But it sometimes poses questions about whose voice the reader of these pages is hearing. I have used the collective "we" when writing about the agency in which most of the contributors work, and when saying things that I believe all or most of us would agree about. But I have used the more personal "I" when offering reminiscences or judgements that other members of the team may not share. If that seems a bit confusing I can only say that it truthfully reflects the cheerfully creative confusion of our collaboration.

I offer warmest thanks to all those who presented cases and discussed drafts at our meetings: Neil Anderson, Charlie Baird, Gerry Burke, Dawn Clarke, Vivien Dance, Mary Doonan, Cathy Douglas, Lindsey Fox Denham, Karen Kerr, Caroline MacAlaster, Maureen Moore, Joan Mulroy, Andrew Park, Maureen Parker, Scott Rorison and Sue Spalton. Scott also wrote Chapter Six, for which he is better equipped than any of us.

Among many others who helped us I particularly want to thank: The Right Honourable Bruce Millan, who chaired the Committee that laid the foundations for the whole scheme we are writing about. Bruce gave me many hours of his time and commented in detail on chapters recording events in which he played a leading role. Councillor Jim Kiddie, who was an active member of Millan's Committee, gave me a lot of help. Shaben Begum and her colleagues at the Scottish Independent Advocacy Alliance, and Nicola Smith and her colleagues at Enable Scotland who work for people with learning disabilities also gave us a lot of help. Hector Mackenzie, a senior official in the Scottish Home and Health Department at the time the advocacy service was built into Scottish law, gave me important insights into these events.

Caroline Airs and her colleagues at GAIN – the Gateshead Advice and Information Network – met with me for a long discussion and commented helpfully on a draft. Professor John Blackie, at Strathclyde University, gave me a perspective that was both warmly humane and legally sophisticated. Donna Strachan and her colleagues at CAPS – the Consultation and Advocacy Promotion Service in Edinburgh – introduced me to an East Coast world that I needed to know more about. Maureen Beaton and Peter Woolfson gave me wise advice about the work of tribunals. Helpfully critical comments on the whole draft or many chapters of it were made by Kay Jones, Joan Mulroy and Rachel Donnison; and colleagues in the Universities of Bristol, Glasgow, Northumbria and York came to seminars to discuss the project with me. I am grateful to all of them.

Finally, Kay Carmichael, my wife, gave me at every stage her usual combination of frank criticism and loving comradeship.

David Donnison
February 2009

Introduction

This book is about advocacy – particularly, but not only, for people who have learning disabilities or mental health difficulties. The practical experience we will draw on comes mainly from Scotland where new and important things have been happening in this field. Here are two examples of the work we will be writing about.

The first is summed up in a big book – a Personal Care Plan, or 'PCP' in the jargon of social work and community nursing. Prepared by an advocate, with help from colleagues in other services, this book is packed with words, pictures, medical prescriptions, names and addresses. It speaks for a young woman – let's call her Sandra – in her mid-twenties.

Sandra has stunted limbs and cannot walk, sit up or feed herself. It takes two people, using a specially made hoist, to lift her from a bed to a chair, or in and out of the swimming pool she visits regularly. She lives at home with her parents. Those who help them to care for her – 32 staff from 13 different agencies see her in a typical week – thought she was unable to speak or to understand anything they said. But her advocate, who works for a local agency, found by listening carefully to her and her parents that she has more than 20 words and sounds that have meanings that she understands pretty well. Indeed her grandmother, who has always loved her dearly, conducts long conversations with her in a language no one else quite understands. Sandra also has hopes and fears, friends she likes to be with, and ambitions for the future.

Her personal care plan explains these and many other things: the foods she can and cannot eat, the movements that hurt her, the medicines she needs and much else. It shows, with photographs, how to lift and move her, and how to take her for a swim.

Equally important, it has brought together 32 nurses, social workers and professional carers – most of whom had never met before – and helped them to get to know each other and to agree on the best ways to help Sandra achieve the things she wants to do. They had to start by breaking out of the hierarchies and specialisms that divide our public service professions and to recognise that they were all equally needed to help the only important person – Sandra herself. They have gained a shared pride in enhancing the life of someone they have come to know. And, because agencies change, their staff move around and Sandra's needs change too, they have to keep in touch and revise her care plan regularly.

Sandra's advocate learnt her skills the hard way – advocating for herself and then for one of her sons. Both have had lifelong and painful physical difficulties. She became a volunteer advocate and later took a paid job with the same agency. Sandra's mother said it was marvellous to find someone who boldly asked for things she would have felt shy about. The family is well supported now by carers and Sandra goes on weekdays to two different day centres. At one of them she met, and immediately recognised, a young man who had been at the special school they had both attended five years earlier. They have become firm friends.

Thanks to her resolute parents, her advocate's help and the team of people they have assembled, Sandra is being recognised as a citizen with rights and needs who must be treated with respect.

Our next example comes from the opposite end of the range of work we will be discussing in this book. It concerns a man with mental health difficulties – let's call him Richard – who had to stay for a long time in hospital.

While in hospital, Richard became quite distressed. No one could understand why until he made contact with one of the workers in the small advocacy unit based in the hospital. She found that he had always had an egg for breakfast, but the hospital kitchen was now providing only toast and cereal. The advocate helped her client to meet and talk with the hospital's clinical dietician and kitchen staff who explained there had been a scare about salmonella poisoning from eggs, which had now therefore been taken off the menu. It was agreed that Richard would have an egg for breakfast once a week – which seemed to satisfy him. Equally important, the advocate believed, was his feeling that he had been able to speak up for himself, had been heard and was treated with respect.

These stories give us a glimpse of important changes now at work in our society – changes in which advocacy plays a part. The old distinction between 'sick' or 'needy' people and the 'normal' people who help and care for them is breaking down. Everyone, no matter what disabilities they may have, can take some control over their lives and achieve some of the things they want to do, if others will allow and help them to do that. The sick and needy have a contribution to make to their own treatment which can be as important as that of trained therapists and helpers: caring for them is a shared task in which the patient or client plays a central part. We all have a right to be treated with respect by those providing the services we depend on. But sometimes each of us will need help in speaking up for ourselves – and particularly when we feel ill, bewildered or frightened. In this book we explore the ways in which these ideas are developing and the contribution that advocacy makes to them.

These stories also pose some of the dilemmas of advocacy. How far should this work go? Was the advocate in our first story doing things that should have been done by staff of other services – or was it her job to teach them how to do these things better in future? How should we measure the success of advocacy? Was it 'success' to get an egg once a week? Or was the greater confidence the patient gained from this achievement more important – therapeutically perhaps? Should advocates be concerned with therapy – or only with helping their clients say whatever they want to say? These are just a few of the questions we will explore in this book.

Both these stories show advocates playing a helpful part in their clients' lives. But that is not how everyone involved in advocacy sees it. While we were writing this book, one of the senior doctors in a hospital where our advocates are working wrote this letter to *The Psychiatric Bulletin*, the journal of the Royal Society set up by his profession. Headlined, 'Right to independent advocacy', his letter says:

> There has been debate over the advantages, if any, of the Mental Health (Scotland) Act, 2003 compared with the Mental Health (Scotland) Act 1984. One of its introductions has been the right for any patient with a mental disorder to access an independent advocate, 'a person who enables the patient to express their views about the decisions being made about their care and treatment by being a voice for the patient and encouraging them to speak out for themselves' (Scottish Executive, 2005). It is noteworthy that this definition of the remit of the advocacy workers precludes the peddling of an anti-psychiatry agenda independent of the wishes of the patient. However, as advocacy workers are employed by organisations not directly funded or run by the Health Board or local authority, their activities are not open to the scrutiny of the Mental Welfare Commission for Scotland, which refers complaints to the commissioning agency.
>
> In principle, independent advocacy for vulnerable people who may have communication difficulties is an excellent idea but in practice it can give people with no health service training the opportunity to pursue a mission to find fault with services regardless of the welfare of the patients. Some advocacy workers misrepresent themselves as working for the

benefit of the patient when their stated purpose is to assist them in expressing views about care and treatment decisions, however harmful or self-destructive these views may be. In contrast, all professionals who make up the multidisciplinary team are employed for the health and welfare of the patient, and are bound by codes of ethics and ever-increasing demands for evidence, accountability and governance.

Unnecessary interference with the patient's confidence in the service being provided undermines the trust which is so often crucial in a therapeutic relationship. Whereas cultivation of suspicion and mistrust can lead to an increase in aggressive and threatening behaviour towards psychiatric staff. When de-escalation efforts by staff are then impeded by advocacy workers, either because they are enjoying the spectacle or because they see it as part of the patient's right to be freely abusive and threatening to staff, their presence moves from being time-consuming to being dangerous. Do other organisations employ skilled professional staff to perform a function and then employ unskilled, untrained staff with a remit to undermine that function and to foster hostility and mistrust? I suspect that businesses interested in profit would not seek to damage consumer confidence and satisfaction by provoking complaints and creating an atmosphere in which morale and productivity will decline.

When time has been spent with someone who has severe communication difficulties to ensure that their views are properly represented it is occasionally possible to see why independent advocacy is considered in principle to be beneficial and why some of the individual practitioners of the function are an asset to the service, usually when they do not adhere too closely to their stated remit. Unfortunately, the damage to therapeutic relationships and interactions, and to the planning and implementation of treatment programmes means that any benefits are greatly outweighed. Until there is a major revision of the Act with significant input from clinicians, it is to be hoped that the aims and methods of advocacy services are redefined to minimise the damage to the health and welfare of the people for whom they are supposed to speak.

[Signed] ———— Consultant Psychiatrist

I had a long talk with the author of this letter, and together we worked out a constructive relationship. He assured me he thought our advocates were doing a good job. We print his letter here, not to fan the embers of anyone's wrath, but because it poses important questions that must be discussed in this book. Should advocates say whatever their clients want them to say? Are there no limits? Or should they confine themselves to advocating what they believe to be in their clients' best interests? Is that their job? Would they know enough to decide what would *be* in their clients' best interests? What training do advocates need and who should provide it (medical schools, law schools, social work schools…)? To whom should the agencies employing them be accountable? How should their competence be measured? All these are among the questions we will discuss.

This is how our book is organised.

In Chapter One we briefly describe the main kinds of advocacy available and trace the origins of these movements. Who created them and what did they hope to achieve?

In Chapter Two we turn to Scotland. Most of the developments traced in the previous chapter are to be seen all over the western world. What was different about Scotland, enabling this country to make a special contribution?

The next three chapters are the 'engine room' of the book, describing and discussing what advocates working in this field do, and posing questions to be discussed in later chapters. The first of the chapters sets out the main branches of the work; the second explores puzzles and dilemmas that arise in the course of it. Both deal with individual clients. Chapter Five describes and discusses advocacy for groups of people and the influence it exerts on the wider community.

Chapter Six, by Scott Rorison, deals with questions of management, starting with the setting up of an advocacy agency, the recruitment of its board and staff, and securing funds for its work, and going on to consider the support its advocates need.

Chapter Seven deals with the work of volunteers in this movement – the training they receive, the contribution they make and the support they need.

Chapter Eight discusses how the work of advocates and the agencies employing them should be evaluated, and to whom they should be accountable.

Chapter Nine discusses 'roadblocks' to the work and the strategies available to agencies that encounter services that completely fail to respond to their clients' needs and rights.

Finally, in Chapter Ten, we look back to the origins of this movement and ask where it is going, what contributions it should make to the wider society, and how it should relate to other strategies for making public service professions more accountable and responsive.

We conclude with some suggestions for further reading, briefly explaining the most interesting features of books in the list.

ONE

Origins of advocacy

To understand advocacy properly – or any other new development in public policy – we should first ask: where did it come from, who created it and what were they trying to achieve? These are historical questions and some readers, who share Henry Ford's view that "history is bunk", may prefer to skip to Chapter Three in which we start explaining what advocates do. Others, realising that advocates help people to speak with greater confidence to power, may want to think more carefully first about the workings of power in our society. That is what this chapter is about. I start with a story from nearly a hundred years ago.

Rule of the gentry

Soon after the First World War a young doctor who had just completed his training to be a Medical Officer of Health (MHO) applied for his first job – to be MOH for a rural district in Kent. Called for interview, he was asked one question only: "Do you hunt?" It happened that he could answer "Yes" to that question and he was promptly appointed. (He told me all this 25 years later.)

Months later, young Dr Metcalfe Brown decided he had to close down the local all-age school, which was plainly unsafe for human use. He was summoned at once to the Hall – home of the local lord of the manor – where the man himself, who was also chairman of his Public Health Committee, boomed at him as he approached: "We only appointed you because you said you would hunt. You've never been with the hounds. And now you want to close my school!" And it was, in a sense, "his" school because, long before, his family had built it.

This must have been a moment when a junior medical officer gratefully recalled that the Victorian legislators who created his service had foreseen this kind of situation. They wrote into their law that those holding the post of Medical Officer of Health could only be sacked with the approval of the Minister in London. Their work would inevitably bring them into conflict from time to time with local landlords, industrialists and other powerful people. No other public official had this protection. It made the MOH the senior local government officer, after the Town Clerk who was the lawyer we would now probably call Chief Executive.

I tell this story because Metcalfe Brown began his career under the old regime, which had for centuries been run by Britain's local gentry, and he was also a forerunner of the regime that was to follow, which brought the public service professions to power.

The old regime can be glimpsed in the novels of Jane Austen. In *Emma*, published in 1816, she describes the lives of the gentry in an English village. All of them depended on cooks, housemaids, coachmen and gardeners to keep their households going and just occasionally we glimpse the existence of these people. But their characters and feelings are never touched on by this marvellously sensitive observer of character and feelings. The gentry – and particularly the local Anglican vicar – are occasionally recorded as performing charitable duties for the deserving poor. But those receiving their charity are never mentioned. The "undeserving poor" are once glimpsed when some gypsy children, supported by their mother and "a great boy", noisily demand alms from two frightened young ladies who are rescued by a passing gentleman. The gypsies are driven out of the village next morning.

George Eliot was an equally famous and more scholarly novelist who had taught herself the science, politics and psychology of her day – reading eight different languages. But her most famous novel, *Middlemarch*, published in 1872, tells us equally little about working-class people. Doctors, three of whom appear in her story, live a rather precarious life, competing to win patients among the gentry and invitations to the great houses.

There were writers who did give working people a central place in their work; most famously Charles Dickens. There were gentry who cared passionately about social justice: people like Josephine Butler, Florence Nightingale, Octavia Hill and Beatrice Webb – great women and leading social reformers. But the average member of the property-owning classes did not regard poor people as citizens who had rights. The brewers, butchers and farmers who served in the horse-riding yeomanry that cut down 18 people, including a woman and her child, and injured hundreds of others when dispersing a crowd of protesters in the Peterloo massacre of 1819 showed what could happen when the gentry became frightened.

The attitudes of the gentry towards the poorest people had not greatly changed when, many years later, the Scottish Christian Social Union held its 1909 conference in the Rothesay Hydro on the Isle of Bute. There a Provost (whom the English would call a Mayor) told his audience that the country's future "depends upon whether the national will applies itself to the cultivation of virile character; whether it reveres the qualities that make for honesty, honour, virtue, sincerity, and truth, or accepts sloth, indolence, cheating, and amusement, as the legitimate rewards of liberty." Another speaker dealt with tramps, dividing them into five groups: "(1) the unemployable, (2) the work-shy class, (3) the in-and-out class [meaning in and out of the workhouse] (4) the old and infirm who wander about and are unemployable, and (5) inebriates". "What we must do", he said, "is to apprehend loafers, beggars, etc., who prey upon society, and commit them to a Labour Colony" (a kind of open prison: he ran one himself.) The Medical Officer for Renfrew said that "tramps and loafers" should "be segregated, and prevented from contaminating others, and more especially from propagating their like". There was much more in the same vein – reminding us that Britain could easily have gone down the path followed later by the Nazis. And we know what the fate of Sandra – briefly described in the Introduction to this book – would then have been.

These 1909 conference papers vividly portray the political assumptions of the local ruling class at this time. They were individualistic and moralistic. They were anxiously concerned about public order. They were locally based, relying for governance on municipal authorities and charities, and hostile to the central state. And they were simplistic in their understanding of economics, assuming that everyone – even older people, those who were sick and those caring for children – could find work and support themselves if only they got off their backsides and tried a bit harder. Their social policies were focused on poverty and its effects; and that encouraged many of them to assume that the poor *were* the problem to be solved.

The gentry challenged

The famous Reports of the Royal Commission on the Poor Laws, which sat between 1905 and 1909, had been published a few weeks before the Rothesay conference. The Minority Report, largely written by Sidney and Beatrice Webb, called for new policies – which took 40 more years to emerge. They argued that the state should create specialist services to meet particular needs (for education, medical care, pensions and so on) for everyone. The Poor Law and its associated charities, which dealt with particular classes of destitute people, should be abolished. That view was contemptuously rejected by speakers at the Christian Social Union's conference.

Working-class people understood pretty well what was going on. *The ragged trousered philanthropists*, written by Robert Tressell who was a working-class man himself, is a novel that makes this clear. Beatrice Webb – still Beatrice Potter at that time – when serving her apprenticeship as social researcher and reformer in the slums of London's East End, went to a demonstration of cookery at which a charitable lady instructed working-class women how to make soup from fish heads which could be bought for a few farthings in the markets at the end of the day. "Any questions?" she asked at the end of her lecture. After a cool pause, a woman at the back asked, "Who ate the fish?"

A generation later, Winifred Holtby in her novel *South Riding*, published in 1936, describes a local government world that was beginning to change. In Yorkshire, a few trade unionists were joining the shopkeepers and genteel ladies who served on the committees. In the coalfields of South Wales, the Labour Party and the National Union of Mineworkers would have wielded more power. But in neither would the public service professions have played a major part. Julian Tudor Hart, a doctor who has written about South Wales at this time, reminds us that most of his colleagues were then still quite poor. One of them, who worked in the poshest practice in Port Talbot, always had to enter his wealthiest patient's home through the tradesmen's entrance. Only when Lord Horder – King George V's doctor – arrived from London to confirm his diagnosis was a doctor admitted through the front door.

Things changed after the Second World War. I still recall vividly the moment, in July 1945, when I heard that the British people had elected their first majority Labour government. I was a midshipman on the bridge of a cruiser steaming across the Indian Ocean through a hot tropical night when the news reached us from our radio operators. Although too young to vote, I had as a schoolboy growing up in the 1930s heard about the fruitless hunger marches of the unemployed to Westminster, the vain attempts of a divided Labour Party to win votes, the lost war against Fascism in Spain, the Japanese continuing rape of China, Mussolini's conquest of Abyssinia, and the terrible things the Nazis were doing to trade unionists, socialists and Jewish people – and I had concluded that the good guys always lose; the bad guys win. At last, the good guys seemed to have won. Was the class war over?

Millions were asking the same question. All across Europe there were countries whose people were hoping for a better world. They wanted peace; they wanted to go home to their wives and children; they wanted opportunities to work at a reasonable wage, decent homes for their families at a rent they could afford, education for their youngsters and medical care when they needed it.

The public service professions come to power

The settlements that politicians and the captains of industry and commerce reached with spokesmen of their working people varied from country to country, but always included an assurance that these basic things would in time be provided. That could only be done through massive interventions by government relying on the public service professions to provide and manage the services that later came to be called 'the welfare state'. The old gentry and their charities survived, but were dethroned, as Sidney and Beatrice Webb and many others had long argued they should be.

When, in 1948, Western Europe's first attempts to build welfare states faltered as slowly recovering economies proved unable to bear the load, the Americans rescued us with Marshall Aid. Their legislators did not particularly like what the Europeans did with their dollars. ("Look at them!" screamed the congressmen in a cartoon by David Low, pointing enraged fingers at a group of frail British pensioners: "Gnashing our own teeth at us!") But they did not want European voters to turn to communist movements backed by the Red Army. The looming presence of that army was a constant reminder to Europe's rulers that there were alternative regimes to which their working people might turn if their needs were neglected.

Gradually the public service professions became the new power in the land. I use that phrase to describe people qualified through higher or further education working in publicly funded organisations providing services that are either free to their users (like education or much of health care) or priced at levels determined by the government for the purpose of meeting needs, not principally for profit (like public housing and prescriptions dispensed for the health service). Their employers may be central or local government, commercial enterprises or voluntary bodies. Each profession has recognised qualifications and an association or institute of some sort that has some responsibility for setting and maintaining standards of practice. They are constantly expanding in numbers. Whether advocates employed to challenge these professions should eventually be included among them is a question we discuss later in this book.

These professions gained increasing power during and after the war. The National Health Service ensured that no fully qualified doctor would henceforth be poor. Aneurin Bevan had to negotiate for months with the top ones before he could persuade them to support his bill, concluding finally that he bought their consent by "stuffing their bloody mouths with gold". When war-damaged houses had been repaired a new building programme was launched, but until 1952 council officials allocated at least 85 per cent of the houses built to those judged to be in greatest need. Development rights were nationalised, so town planners and building controllers decided where houses could be built and what size they would be. Food was distributed under an official rationing system that was more severe than anything experienced during the war. Everyone, rich and poor, had to have their ration book. (And the poor became healthier that ever before because everyone had much the same diet.) Metcalfe Brown – who had by the 1950s become Professor of Public Health at the University of Manchester – was teaching the next generation of Medical Officers of Health that they should never call their committees together without writing the minutes of the meeting beforehand. "But take care not to let committee members see them until afterwards."

All these professions were subject, ultimately, to democratically elected politicians in central or local government. That was the theory justifying their authority; and it worked pretty well for the people who had the backing of large numbers of voters. Not so well for minority ethnic groups and for Catholics in Protestant parts of Northern Ireland.

As the years went by, rationing relented and the private sector of the economy revived. But, while politicians might decide what the nation could afford in various sectors of its public economy, their programmes were shaped by a power structure dominated by the most powerful groups within the public service professions. Thus Bevan had hoped for a health service that would meet the daily needs of ordinary patients, modelled on what was already developing in the mining constituencies he knew so well. But what we got was a service dominated by hospitals in which the consultants in the most prestigious specialisms dominated hospital governors – "guaranteeing", as Tudor Hart has said, "that essential but unromantic specialities like geriatrics and psychiatry stayed safely at the bottom of the staff ladder and the end of the resource queue."[1]

Within the school system it was many years – long after other countries had reached similar conclusions – before the dominance of the selective grammar schools and their university backers could be challenged and a comprehensive system began to take shape.

When the time came for the nation to face the need for a massive expansion of its universities, the Robbins Committee, to which the question was referred, brushed aside the arguments of those who wanted new universities built in the centres of industrial cities within reach of the thousands of working people who had never had a chance of higher education. Most of the new ones were built in somewhat decayed cathedral towns, the kind of places dons like to live in – pretty places from which they could travel to London and back for professional and political meetings within a day.

The new regime treated working-class people better than the old one had done – particularly by ensuring for many years that there was full employment. Opportunities for education, housing and health care were gradually transformed, and there was a big expansion in the array of services to which people had legal rights – rights to secondary education, health care and social security benefits, for example. Great though the power of their officials was, these professionals were not also the employers, landlords, magistrates or priests of those who depended on them, as the gentry had often been. They could more readily be challenged; so advocacy on behalf of the challengers became possible too.

The services of the welfare state were steadily expanded and improved by an unspoken but powerful alliance between the professions that made their living by working in them and the better-organised working people who depended heavily on them for health care, pensions, housing and the education of their children. Both were to be seen in local meetings of the Labour Party up and down the country where skilled workers, trade unionists and council tenants sat alongside teachers, social workers, local government officers and the like.

But the poorest people – those most likely to be excluded from the mainstream of society by poverty, sickness, disability and discrimination of various kinds – were often unemployed or unable to work, and therefore not represented by trade unions. For years, while chairing the Supplementary Benefits Commission, which had a responsibility for Britain's means-tested social benefits, I attended the annual conferences of the Trades Union Congress. There one would hear cogent arguments for better health and safety at work, better state retirement pensions – benefits for organised workers. But rarely was anything said about supplementary benefits, or what we would now call Jobseeker's Allowance, or benefits for lone parents.

There are of course trade unionists and socialists who have devoted their lives to helping the poorest people without asking whether they belong to a union or a political party. Joe Kenyon was one such campaigner for social justice, as a miner, a trade union official, later in other work and finally as a pensioner. His marvellous book, *A passion for justice*,[2] tells the story. But, too often, the poorest people have found themselves neglected and excluded by the public service professions, their unions and professional associations.

David Bull, working for the Child Poverty Action Group as one of their volunteer advocates in the 1970s, found that when he put up notices in social security offices informing claimants about their rights these were often torn down by staff. Managers told him, when he offered to set up advice counters in their offices to help claimants, that this would "cause trouble with staff side" – the civil service trade unions. Many years later, Stewart Brandon, in his vivid book, *The invisible wall*,[3] tells the story of a boy with severe physical and learning difficulties who was happily educated in a mainstream primary school where other pupils welcomed and supported him – their own performance improving as a result. But, when his parents tried to get a place for him in the local secondary school, with the agreement of its head – in a local authority that officially favoured mainstream education for such children – it was the staff unions who compelled their governors to withdraw the offer by threatening strike action.

The professions disempowered

By the 1970s, changes working their way through western economies were altering their class structures. At the end of the Second World War about two thirds of Britain's labour force worked with their hands – mainly in manufacturing industries, transport and mining – and two thirds lived in rented housing – mainly belonging to private landlords. More than two thirds of our children went to schools in which the educational ladder petered out at the age of 14. This was the massive working class. They did not all vote Labour; but if they wanted someone to speak for them to authority it was to their unions, their politicians and the mass media they naturally turned, not to lawyers, the courts or voluntary bodies whom they regarded as classic representatives of the middle class.

But manufacturing industries and other employers of skilled manual labour were declining. More and more people found they could only get a decent home by buying their own houses. Trade union membership and support for the traditional labour movement also declined. Britain, which had been growing slowly more equal in its distribution of income and wealth until the early 1970s, began – slowly at first, and then very rapidly in the late1980s – to grow more unequal.

The alliance for progressive reform, which had carried forward the development of the welfare state, was breaking up. The potential support for higher taxes and better social programmes, which in the early post-war years had been highest among poorer people and lowest among the rich, now took on a U shape – lower among the middle third than among those richer or poorer. These 'Middle England' people had to be listened to because it was the swing voters among them who made and unmade governments.

Margaret Thatcher was the first major politician to recognise the political implications of the new society that was emerging. Through changes in taxation and benefits her governments transferred funds from poorer to richer people on a massive scale, without, at first, provoking any serious resistance. The public service professions were disempowered, along with their power bases in local government, the unions and the universities. The government no longer felt it needed royal commissions, advisory committees and committees of inquiry. Their reports on public policy had been formulated after a lengthy process of gathering and sifting evidence from experts of every kind. But their conclusions were often shaped with an eye to the interests of the public service professions that furnished so many of their members and witnesses – professions that would eventually have to put their recommendations into practice.

Henceforth, new ideas for policy were fed directly into government by politically committed 'think tanks' and 'policy advisers'. (That's how we got council tax – and now secondary school 'academies'.) Kenneth Clark, when Secretary of State for Health, introduced the biggest changes the National Health Service had experienced since it was founded. Whereas spokesmen of the British Medical Association, the teaching hospitals and the royal colleges had held up Bevan's original bill through months of negotiation, their successors learned of Clark's reforms along with the rest of us, from the newspapers and the *Today* programme. The professions marched in protest against cuts in their services under the banners of their unions and professional associations. But their tenants, pupils and patients, the social security claimants and social work clients, did not march at their side.

Preparing the ground for advocacy

By the late 1960s, a new generation of radicals had come to recognise that they could not simply rely on parties of the Left or the professions running the welfare state to put social injustices right. They formed a growing range of independent pressure groups offering advice and support to deprived communities, families and individuals, and mounting larger campaigns at local and national levels. The Child Poverty Action Group, founded in 1965, was one of the first. Shelter, campaigning about homelessness, began the following year. Other groups that were concerned with the rights and needs of women, lone parents, minority ethnic groups, asylum seekers, pensioners, gays and lesbians, particular deprived neighbourhoods and people with a steadily growing variety of illnesses and disabilities followed.

These groups were not a united movement. They competed with each other for public attention and for resources. But they shared important and fundamental ideas: the idea that all people have the same basic human rights and that every citizen is entitled to be treated with respect; the idea that everyone – no matter how disadvantaged they may appear to be – has a contribution to make to society that they should be enabled to offer; the idea that human needs can be most effectively met when those who have these needs collaborate on terms of mutual respect with those expert in helping them; and the idea that many 'handicaps' are not inherent in people's condition. They are created by society's failure to respond to their needs and recognise their rights. A new climate of opinion was emerging, fostering new ways of providing professional services and new ways of conducting politics. All this provided fertile ground for the development of advocacy – a reinvention of features of trade union and legal practice organised in ways that would help people who usually had no union and no lawyer to speak for them.

This was not just a British phenomenon. The European Court of Human Rights had, since the 1950s, increasingly compelled the British to recognise they were laggards in recognising human rights in many fields. Perhaps lawyers and the law had a part to play in creating a fairer society? Our own Human Rights Act of 1998 imported European ideas, enabling British citizens to seek such rights without having to journey to the continent. Prisoners have recently compelled the Home Office to rebuild its jails by arguing successfully in court that slopping out is an infringement of their basic human rights. Lawyers are moving into the human rights debate in growing numbers.

Meanwhile other developments have demystified and discredited traditional authorities of various kinds, and emboldened people to challenge them. Consumer movements that began in the US have spread to other countries, enabling people collectively to exert pressure on those in the public and private sectors to improve the goods and services they offer us. Growing use of the internet sends more patients to their doctors' surgeries convinced they have 'Googled' the cause of their distress and found the appropriate treatment they should demand for it. Recurring scandals of sexual abuse by clergy and by staff of residential institutions, and the growing willingness of service users to challenge professional staff and sometimes to demand compensation in court – all these have played their parts in preparing the ground for advocacy.

Unresolved questions

But the regime that is now emerging poses many unanswered questions. The welfare states created by western nations after the Second World War had some clearly understood aims and principles. William Beveridge, in his famous wartime report, set out the practical implications of the Webbs' vision. Modern democracies, it was widely assumed, would grow slowly but steadily more equal. Their citizens should be entitled to opportunities for work at reasonable pay, decent services for education and health care at points in their lives when they needed these things, cash benefits for their children, and an adequate income during periods of sickness and unemployment and finally in retirement. All these had to be provided by government services manned by the growing public service professions. Means-tested benefits for the poorest people, it was assumed, would only be needed in a small number of exceptional and probably temporary cases. We had a long way to go to attain this utopian vision. But at least we *had* a vision and thought we knew where we were heading.

It was a vision in which citizenship, comradeship and the collective responsibility that a society's members have for each other played central parts. Many of those responsibilities would be carried by the public service professions, whose members would have a public service 'ethos' or morality that would be different from those of the profit-driven market place.

What we now have is a society that has grown much more unequal over the past generation. Its public sector is supposed to offer growing opportunities for choice to people who are regarded as individual customers of services provided by a mixed array of public, commercial and charitable agencies competing against each other. Our housing is mainly owner-occupied – meaning that most of it belongs to banks, building societies and other lenders to which we pay money that may eventually entitle us to call these places our own. Only a minority of people buy their own education and medical care – but these minorities are growing. Frail people entitled to care provided by the state are encouraged to use direct payments that make them the choosers and employers of those who care for them. Meanwhile we make growing use of means-tested benefits – far more than other countries do – to support those who struggle to get by in these markets.

There are clearly some good things about the new regime. If the staff of public services think of those who depend on them as 'customers', they may be more inclined to treat them efficiently and courteously. But, if our role as citizens – with the collective responsibilities that brings – is replaced by that of individual customers there will be losses too. Many forms of care call for close team work between different professions concerned with the same client. (Sandra, described in our Introduction, is a vivid example, served by 32 people from 13 different agencies.) Will competition between these agencies make team work easier or harder? And what happens if public service professions abandon their responsibility to decide priorities between different needs and different clients, and simply give priority to the most demanding 'customers'?

As advocacy develops, we have to ask whether it will strengthen the idea of citizenship or further weaken it? Will it help to create a more equal society or further exclude the people who don't have an advocate to speak for them? These are some of the questions we consider later in this book.

Meanwhile, in recent months, the ideology of the profit-driven market place, which many had thought to be the only political philosophy in town, has been devastatingly discredited. No one expects that we will go back to the Old Left's reliance on the state. So there is a vacuum at the heart of western thinking about governance. A book about advocacy offers too small a stage for exploring these large questions. But we will have to bear them in mind when we come to consider the future development of advocacy and the part it may play on the larger stage.

Advocacy for people with mental disorders

The time has come to focus on advocacy that helps people who have learning disabilities or mental health difficulties. There are good books by the Brandons, by Dorothy Atkinson, by Rick Henderson and Mike Pochin, and by others – briefly introduced in our final notes on Further Reading – that trace the development of this work, which is why the story will only be briefly summarised here. Others have written well about advocacy for particular groups of clients: deprived children or victims of domestic violence, for example. But few have said much about the broader political movements that have helped to bring advocacy into being, or about the kind of society that advocacy may be helping to create. We have to think about those things too. Advocacy conducted only for its own sake – to 'win' cases for the few clients who happen to get this help, without any coherent vision of the future – will be less creative than it should be.

The story of advocacy for people with mental disorders has been traced back to John Clare, the 'peasant poet' who spent the last 27 years of his life in asylums until he died in 1864. He was more witness than advocate. John Perceval was perhaps the first real advocate in this field. Son of the Prime Minister who was assassinated by a mentally disturbed man in the House of Commons in 1812, he had a breakdown himself nearly 20 years later. Although he was discharged from his asylum after a year, he devoted much of the rest of his life to campaigning on behalf of people who suffered the kind of treatment he had experienced there. With others, he founded The Alleged Lunatic's Friend Society and became its Honorary Secretary. David Brandon describes him as the "great grandfather of the English mental illness service reform movements".

The huge array of asylums that grew up in England were, in the main, a Victorian creation. In 1827 there were only nine, with just over a thousand patients in all. By 1890 there were 66, with 53,000 patients. Residential institutions were the Victorians' main instrument for dealing with destitute people, neglected children, 'the deranged', and anyone else thought to be dangerous or unable to fend for themselves.

The terrors of the First World War drove many – officers, as well as their men – into mental breakdowns, often called 'shell shock' at that time. This helped people to recognise that these men were ill, not just cowards or weaklings. The Second World War had a similar impact, at a time when doctors were beginning to develop more effective forms of treatment. The National Health Service brought about a great expansion in psychiatry after 1948. Between the wars, the pharmaceutical industry had begun to produce behaviour-controlling drugs on a scale that is still growing. These made other forms of treatment possible, not only in asylums but out in the community as well. They also conferred medical status and growing power on psychiatrists.

Women and the lowest-paid workers gained the biggest increases in wages during the war. With labour scarcities continuing afterwards, thanks to the first peacetime full employment ever achieved, it became increasingly difficult and expensive to run asylums. Like other residential institutions, they had always relied heavily on low-paid women to keep them going.

Meanwhile, along with better opportunities for paid work, more generous social security benefits and the continuing growth of subsidised housing, the new drugs made it possible to get more people out of hospitals – people who had often been warehoused there only because they would otherwise have been destitute and homeless.

The Royal Commission on Mental Illness and Mental Deficiency, which sat from 1954 till 1957, reappraised the whole field. Its report led to the 1959 Act which brought about massive changes for England and Wales. Scotland's Act followed next year. In 1961 Enoch Powell, Minister of Health, called for a halving within 15 years of the 150,000 beds then occupied in mental hospitals. That was achieved, but without creating an adequate alternative system to provide care in the community.

Backed by a growing concern about human rights, advocacy on behalf of marginalised groups became a growing practice all across the western world. The movements launched for women, consumers and minority ethnic groups – most of them taking off first in the US – offered aggressive, rights-based models for political thought and action that were later taken up by British people concerned about mental disorders. Their writings often neglect to remind us of the support they were given by a succession of distinguished psychiatrists: humane therapists, great teachers and original thinkers. They included: John Bowlby, who stressed the central part played by consistent affection and good parenting in our mental health; his colleague, Donald Winnicott, a great child psychiatrist and teacher; Maxwell Jones, who created a therapeutic community in his hospital, Dingleton, where patients and all grades of staff met to work together on equal terms; and R.D. Laing, who challenged his colleagues to listen more carefully to their patients, to look at their whole family setting, and to intervene as little and as humanely as possible.

Advocacy for people with mental disorders began to emerge as an organised practice in Britain in the 1970s. The growth of Mental Health Review Tribunals, set up in England under the 1959 Act and later strengthened by the Mental Health Act of 1983, provided a forum for the practice of advocacy by lawyers and lay people who became expert in this branch of the law. Independent groups mobilising to support patients were usually founded by their relatives. The National Schizophrenia Fellowship – now SANE (Schizophrenia a national emergency) – and Mencap (speaking for parents and carers of people with learning disabilities) were two of the first and still among the best known.

In the 1980s a number of health professionals who had themselves had breakdowns and a spell in hospital wrote about their experiences – another challenge to the stigma of 'madness'.

As patients, now returning more quickly to the community, came home in better shape to cope with the world, groups of them spoke up more confidently. They were usually local groups, often hospital-based, working with sympathetic junior staff and giving them encouragement and 'space' to do innovative things. But at no point did advocates get secure, long-term funding to provide a genuinely independent service. As a result, these projects were always insecure. Those run by service users tended to burn out eventually, and those collaborating closely with staff tended to become co-opted by the professionals and to lose their vigorous independence.

Most of the professionals had not grasped – indeed, some of the best academics writing about the mental health services had not grasped – that an essentially political problem lay at the heart of these services: a problem of power. There were power struggles between the professions involved: psychiatrists of different kinds, nurses, social workers and others. Meanwhile, people with learning disabilities or mental health difficulties were not treated with the respect accorded to citizens who had other kinds of illness. That was not because the professionals were generally uncaring or brutal – although some of them were. It was because the broader society, in whose culture the professions were rooted, was uncaring – frightened even – about these most excluded people.

This book is not about yet another group of workers claiming to do good things for people and bidding to join the public service professions. It is about a movement bidding to change that world.

Different kinds of advocacy

There is no single thing that the term 'advocacy' describes. The whole field of work is now immensely varied. These are the main forms of advocacy that people with mental health difficulties or learning disabilities may encounter.

1   *Informal or natural advocates*: there will always be people to whom others in trouble with authorities of various kinds turn for advice and support – men and women of courage and considerable experience who may have no formal qualifications of any kind. Before turning to others we should always ask: is such a person available? Can any professional do better?

2   *Political advocacy* by elected representatives at all levels of government who have always devoted much of their time to helping their constituents to gain their rights. This is an ancient and honourable

tradition. But new advocacy movements would not have developed if it had been sufficient.

3   *Advocacy by professionals for their own patients or clients*, in which doctors, nurses, social workers or others in the public service professions do their best to ensure that those they care for get the best treatment available from others with authority to give or withhold it – a practice complicated by the fact that the professionals also have potentially conflicting obligations to other patients and to their own colleagues.

4   *Self-advocacy*, in which patients, social work clients and others with particular needs are enabled to speak up for themselves, with varying amounts of support. This obviously works best for those who are reasonably fit, competent, confident and speak good English.

5   *Peer advocacy*, in which people are supported by advocates who have had experiences similar to their own and have come through them with some success. These advocates have expertise gained from their own experience. But it will be important to ensure that they speak for their clients and are not still fighting their own battles.

6   *Parents' and carers' advocacy* for the people they are looking after. Since they probably know the patient or client better than anyone else, they are also experts who must be listened to. But their role may be complicated by the fact that the needs and views of different people in a family or household will sometimes conflict.

7   *Citizen advocacy*, in which an individual volunteer gives long-term support to one person – their 'partner'. Started in Sweden in the 1950s and later taken up in the US, this was a movement originally set up by parents whose children had learning disabilities to provide answers to the question: what will happen to him or her after I am gone? It may amount to befriending rather than advocacy; and if volunteers lose heart or move away their partners may feel badly let down.

8   *Professional advocacy*, conducted for their clients by lawyers and other professionally trained advocates. These professionals have special skills to offer. But some people have warned that this may insert yet another layer of bureaucracy to which patients and clients are subordinated.

All these kinds of work may be conducted individually, or among groups of people with similar needs who support each other and may collectively approach the authorities to seek changes in the services they depend on. A mixed strategy is often followed in which most of the work is individual but occasional group meetings take place. The work may be based in hospitals, day centres or shop-front offices; or it may be done from advocates' homes. It may be done by paid staff or unpaid volunteers, or by a mixture of the two.

There is a tendency in some of the literature about particular kinds of advocacy for its authors to claim the moral high ground for their favourite form of it, and to dismiss others as inferior. Our standpoint is that each form has its own strengths and weaknesses, and each can be very helpful. We should not discourage people from working in any of these ways.

9   None of these categories exactly describes the form of advocacy that this book mainly deals with. This may be called 'issue-based advocacy – mainly for individuals'. What exactly this means will be explained in the chapters that follow.

Notes

[1] Julian Tudor Hart, *The political economy of health care*, Bristol, The Policy Press, 2006.

[2] Joe Kenyon, *A passion for justice: The stories of Joe Kenyon*, Nottingham, Trent Editions, 2003.

[3] Stewart Brandon, *The invisible wall: Niki's fight to be included*, Hesketh Bank, Parents With Attitude, 1997.

TWO

Scotland gives a lead

Questions posed

The story we have told thus far is typical of the way a social reform takes shape. First there are economic and social changes: in this case, labour scarcities which make hospital and residential care more expensive, new drugs which make them less necessary, more jobs, more subsidised housing and more generous social benefits to help sick and disabled people survive in the community. The same things were happening in every western country. In most of them the numbers in mental hospitals peaked between 1965 and 1975. In Scotland there has been a dramatic reduction since then in the numbers of patients in these hospitals, but slightly more are entering them – most of them only for short periods. Difficult decisions had to be made about the small minority of these patients who had to be treated under compulsion, whether in hospitals or in the community. These decisions were taken by sheriffs' courts, which dealt with piles of papers and rarely saw the patients themselves.

Thus economic and social changes create new problems but also offer hope for better solutions: particularly, in this case, better care in the community for all sorts of people who no longer have to be confined in hospitals.

Also playing a part in the story were social and political changes, such as the growth of an increasingly well-informed and litigious population, more inclined to question authority. Complaints about health care reaching the UK's General Medical Council numbered 1,087 in the year 1991/92. Thirteen years later, in 2004/05, they had risen more than fourfold to 4,452. A growing array of increasingly confident voluntary bodies had grown up to speak for various groups with special needs. Meanwhile, the whole idea of human rights was spreading, and powerful movements were demanding equal rights for women, for minority ethnic groups, for gays and lesbians and for others.

In Scotland, as elsewhere, groups speaking for people with mental illnesses or learning disabilities – together we will call them mental disorders – came fairly late in the growing queue of those demanding a response from the state to their needs and rights: late and with less political clout. Like others, they set up voluntary bodies providing information, advice and advocacy. Thus, by the end of the 20th century, there was a growing array of voluntary bodies engaged in advocacy in many fields – usually coupled with other kinds of help. And they were getting growing support from public funds. The scene was set for a growth of such services that could play a modest but important part within a larger set of political changes. Their shared aim was to gain recognition for the rights of people depending on public services to be treated with respect, to enable them to play an active part in choosing and planning their own treatment, and to lead as independent a life as possible. Many of those taking these initiatives recognised that their work needed a political cutting edge, questioning the balance of power between providers and users of public services.

But difficult questions had still to be answered. Would separate advocacy services develop for people with different needs – those with physical or learning disabilities, housing tenants, children cared for by the state and so on? Or would one service develop to help anyone who walked through its doors? How would responsibilities for managing and funding such services be divided between central government, local government and voluntary bodies? Would they be organised on a national or a local basis? Once publicly funded, how independent could advocates be? Which groups and what needs should have priority?

Developments of this sort, posing similar questions, had taken place throughout the western world, without leading to the creation of a general right to independent advocacy or any reliable nationwide service to provide it. So why did Scotland give a lead in setting up such a service? Why did it focus particularly on the needs of people with mental disorders? And what answers is Scotland giving to the questions we have posed? If we understood these things better we would be better placed to understand the scope, the dilemmas and the potential future of a service of this kind – issues that will be explored in greater depth in later chapters.

While this book focuses particularly on Scotland we will also be using the opportunities this small country's experiment offers us to learn lessons that may be useful elsewhere. If they are to create similar services other countries will face similar dilemmas.

Political response

Economic and social changes prepare the ground for reforms. But it takes people and political leadership to decide what to do and bring about change.

When a Scottish Parliament was recreated in 1999 it was able to deal with about 15 major pieces of legislation each year in place of the two or three Scottish Acts that the Westminster Parliament had previously found time for. But most of the powers of the state remained either with the Westminster Parliament – for taxation, defence, social security and so on – or with local government, which was responsible for most aspects of education, planning, social work and so on. Health was the policy field that gave Members of the Scottish Parliament their biggest budget, their biggest media coverage and their biggest postbags; and in a country with one of the worst health records in the developed world they had plenty of work to do.

One of the first papers produced by the Scottish Executive – Scotland's government – was *The same as you?*, published in 2000. It was designed to improve the lives of people with learning disabilities. Its 29 recommendations included proposals for social work and health partnerships, better local area coordination, person-centred plans of the kind briefly described in our Introduction, more 'meaningful' day services that would involve and consult their users and respond to their aspirations and needs, better opportunities for education and employment – and independent advocacy.

There would clearly be a need for a new Mental Health Act to replace the Act of 1984. In fact, there had not been a major reappraisal of policies in this field since the great Act of 1959 – 1960 in Scotland –40 years earlier.

The Scots set about this task in the traditional British way – by appointing a Committee of Inquiry. This had started work before the new Parliament was created in 1999. Scottish Office ministers chose for it a chairman whose name would make it clear that this issue was going to be taken seriously. The Right Honourable Bruce Millan had long been a Glasgow Labour MP, had held ministerial and commissioner posts in the Westminster and European governments, and had been Secretary of State for Scotland in the Westminster Parliament. He was also on the board of the Scottish Association for Mental Health. He was respected in the Scottish political and mental health worlds and knew his way around them. He started by insisting that his terms of reference be revised to give his Committee a bit more elbowroom, removing "public safety" from his brief and replacing this phrase with "the public interest". He assembled an able Committee of 16 members who included at least two people who had extensive experience as users of mental health services. In Hilary Patrick, Millan had an able and sympathetic lawyer who had specialised in this field. These people were to become particularly important when the question of advocacy was broached.

The Committee travelled around Scotland to meet and talk with staff of the health and social work services, lawyers and the police, voluntary agencies, pressure groups, service users and people caring for relatives with mental disorders. Two large-scale consultations were held with people from these and other fields, and a record of their discussions was sent back to them, inviting further comments. The Committee was not just 'inquiring', as a professor or a 'think tank' might have done. It was raising expectations for reform and helping to build a movement to support it.

There was already an extensive network of voluntary bodies working in this field with a lot of support from government – groups eager to play their part in such a movement. Officials in the Home and Health Department encouraged these groups to get together and helped them to gain a voice that had to be listened to. They formed a consortium, which led to the creation of a larger grouping of about a dozen of the bigger agencies, named Advocacy 2000. This in its turn became the much larger Scottish Independent Advocacy Alliance whose purpose is "to promote, support and defend" independent advocacy in Scotland.

In 1997 the Department had published *Advocacy: A guide to good practice*, a report aimed particularly at health boards and local government to encourage them to make better and more consistent use of advocates. The Department persuaded its ministers to take advocacy seriously – not an easy matter when the first of them was a man who had been a senior surgeon. It got him and his successors to come to conferences of the voluntary agencies working in this field and listen to their spokesmen.

One of these officials – Hector Mackenzie, in the Health Planning and Quality Unit of the Home and Health Department – had tried to persuade his colleagues in other departments of the Executive who were responsible for education, housing, childcare and other matters to contribute to a joint budget that would fund advocacy for users of every public service. It would have been a bold and imaginative step – but they declined the challenge. Mackenzie's challenge is a reminder that it was a historical accident that a right to free and independent advocacy took off first in the field of mental disorder. It might have begun anywhere; and it may yet penetrate everywhere.

The Millan Committee visited England to learn from experience south of the border – looking particularly at the tribunal system that the English had set up to take over much of the work still done by courts in Scotland. England had set up an inquiry of its own, but it seemed a less happy operation. There was conflict within the committee and the Scots felt their English colleagues would be restricted in what they could say by the requirements imposed on them by their terms of reference. They had to report both to the Health Department and to the Home Office – the latter wielding greater power. The minister speaking for the Home Office's concerns about public order and social control seemed constantly worried about the headlines that might appear in tabloid media.

The Scots had recognised that the problems posed by the tiny minority of dangerously violent patients had to be confronted. They did this by appointing a separate committee for the purpose, chaired by Judge Maclean, which worked fast on its more limited task and got its report out first. The Maclean and Millan Committees had the same secretary, Colin Mackay, who did most of their drafting. He was an experienced lawyer who had previously worked for ENABLE Scotland, an umbrella group speaking for people with learning disabilities.

A far-seeing report

The Millan Committee's report *New directions*, published in 2001, appears at first sight to deal mainly with the legal and administrative arrangements required to bring about the closure of old mental hospitals and the transfer of their patients to 'the community' – whatever that might prove to mean. The Committee was equally concerned with users of the mental health services who were living in their own homes. They wrote only one chapter on advocacy – both 'individual' and 'collective' – which produced only seven recommendations. (This contrasts with the 11 dealing with sexual abuse of patients and 14 on the 'named persons' that patients should be entitled to appoint to speak for them.) But closer reading reveals that advocacy was an important thread running through the whole document.

The Committee called for a new system of specialist tribunals, modelled on the English version – but 'properly resourced' – to deal with cases where patients may be subject to compulsion because they disagree with their doctors or are not capable of following their advice. These tribunals would have a lawyer in the chair, flanked by a doctor working in the mental health field and a third member who should have relevant professional experience – as a social worker or an occupational therapist, for example; or they might be someone with 'personal experience as a carer or user of mental health services' (not groups that have put in much of an appearance so far).

Many of the patients coming out of hospitals would be leaving what had for years been their home and workplace. Some would have little knowledge of the world outside its gates or the services available to help them there. Although the new tribunals would actually meet patients and listen to them, their decisions could be appealed to the courts on grounds of law and procedure so they would have to work in fairly formal ways. Thus many patients would need the help of an advocate of some kind.

That conclusion would in any case have followed from the basic 'principles' set out in the Introduction to the report. When patients have to be cared for, there should be "compulsion only where absolutely necessary". Doctors should always seek "the least restrictive alternative" (R.D. Laing had been heard at last). "[F]ormal rights", the Committee said "are not, in themselves, enough. People must feel able to use these rights. It is a matter of concern that so few patients at the moment feel able to appeal against detention ... formal rights to challenge decisions are not a substitute for involving the patient as fully as possible in decisions about his or her care. We therefore recommend greater access to advocacy ... the Principles of *Equality* and *Respect for Diversity*" (their capitals and italics) are fundamental to this philosophy.

"We would also hope that a new Act might help to reduce the stigma which, unfortunately, through ignorance and prejudice, still attaches to mental disorder. This is all the more unfortunate since most of us at some time in our lives will be affected, directly or indirectly, through mental illness in our family or among our friends." (Such sentences should be carved into the walls of every hospital dealing with mental disorders.)

In its first chapter the Committee says that: "The current Act [passed in 1984] has been more concerned with buildings than people". It "reflects an assumption that people with severe mental disorders will require care in a hospital setting. This does not reflect modern practice." The dominant part long played by residential institutions in our social policies – the response to extreme needs of every kind invented by our Victorian forbears – was at last coming to an end, except in our prisons.

The Committee set forth its principles for advocacy thus: "advocacy means: enabling people as far as possible to make informed choices about, and to remain in control of, their own health care". Its aims are:"To promote respect for rights, freedoms and dignity of vulnerable people, both individually and collectively.To ensure people receive the care or services to which they are entitled and which they wish to receive … To enhance people's autonomy … To assist people to live as independently as possible and in the least restrictive environment …To help protect disadvantaged people from abuse and exploitation." No better description has been given.

The Committee's chapter on advocacy services is punctuated by the following recommendations.

1 The Mental Health Act [which they hoped to see before long] should give a right to all mental health service users to obtain access to an advocate [not just those subject to compulsion or those in hospitals] …
2 There should be an obligation on service providers to inform service users about the availability of advocacy services, and to take steps to ensure that the user has an advocate if the user so wishes …
3 There should be a joint duty on health boards and local authorities to ensure that advocacy services are available …
4 The duty to ensure that advocacy is of a satisfactory standard should fall on the commissioning services …
5 The Scottish Executive should give consideration to what steps it should take to provide advocacy for carers.
6 There should be a statutory obligation on service providers to provide support services to collective advocacy groups as required …
7 There should be a statutory obligation on service providers to recognise collective advocacy groups, whether in hospital or elsewhere, as a legitimate voice of service users and involve them in decisions on service development and policy.

After long debate, the Committee came down in favour of a locally based advocacy service, not a single, Scotland-wide organisation. It should be provided by voluntary agencies that would be obliged to shed other work they might be doing in order to assure their independence and avoid conflicts of interest. Collective advocacy by groups of service users should be supported and listened to; individual advocacy would not be enough. Meanwhile, the already existing Mental

Welfare Commission should have stronger powers to visit hospitals and discharge patients whenever they saw fit. This too, the Committee pointed out, would strengthen the case for a right to advocacy.

How did they do it?

How did Bruce Millan's Committee come to such radical conclusions? Being free from the oppressive power of the Home Office certainly helped. So did the experience and conviction of Scottish people working in the field of mental disorder, and the Committee's willingness to learn from them. The commitment of a few officials in the Department of Health who had long believed in advocacy and knew the field well also played an important part. Equally important was the influence of committee members and witnesses who had themselves been users of the mental health services and still had close links with groups of service users in many parts of Scotland.

Jim Kiddie was one of the members of the Millan Committee. He had been a health service manager and an active trade unionist. When managing a 700-bed hospital for people with learning disabilities, he had recognised that many of them 'were no different from me' and, with help from medical colleagues, set about rehabilitating them and getting them discharged with support from housing, social work and other services. Later he headed Grampian Region's mental health services, which, he felt, allowed stresses to develop among its senior staff that led to several breakdowns and a suicide.

Jim eventually collapsed under the strain, made an unsuccessful suicide attempt and spent some three years in mental hospitals in various Scottish cities. There he had experiences that too many patients would find familiar: electric shock treatment from which his memory has never fully recovered; massive doses of drugs whose purposes and side effects were not explained; occupational therapy of humiliating kinds, demanding muscular dexterity he would never have been capable of; nurses who offered to buy drugs off him for resale on the street; and nurses who showed no respect for their patients' sexuality. Finally he also received some effective and kind treatment, secured his discharge and then faced the equally daunting task of living on his own 'in the community'. For a while he was homeless, sleeping on other people's floors. These experiences, which sound like a story from some Victorian madhouse, took place in the 1990s in some of Scotland's biggest cities – at the hands of professionally trained people.

Jim eventually rebuilt his confidence, skills and a circle of friends, and played a leading part in supporting and advocating for patients in the big Royal Edinburgh Hospital. He is now an active town councillor in Aberdeen. He even rediscovered the wife who had divorced him 20 years earlier – introduced to her by their son – and they were remarried. By being prepared to tell others about his experiences – with honesty and some anger but without self-pity – he must have helped many people to throw off the humiliating stigma of mental illness. By campaigning for the development of free and independent advocacy for people in similar situations he will help to make such experiences less common in future. He would add, however, that any progress he and other service users have achieved always depended on the support of humane and progressive doctors, nurses and other professionals – of whom he found many in the Royal Edinburgh Hospital.

Another member of the Millan Committee – Graham Morgan – was the Advocacy Development Officer for HUG (the Highland Users' Group). Bruce Millan appreciated the meticulous way in which he reported the, sometimes conflicting, views of his Group about proposals under discussion in the Committee. Graham and Jim worked together to keep advocacy on the agenda. They understood professional power and the ways in which it can be abused.

Making a law

When a Royal Commission or Committee of Inquiry publishes its report, its leading members travel from one conference to another to present their findings to various professions who may have to do something about them. But after a few months they have to return to their normal work and are forgotten. The officials who helped to write their report and do some of the research that went into it are usually moved at once to some quite different branch of their department where they become far too busy with other things to press for action on the proposals they helped to draft. This is how bureaucracies protect themselves from external influences. They may have little choice; by then a new government may have been elected which has no sympathy for the reforms proposed by a committee they did not appoint.

But in Scotland there was no change of government. The new Minister, Susan Deacon, and her colleagues gave strong support to the Millan Committee's proposals and a group of Members of the Scottish Parliament (MSPs) was set up to carry them forward. Bruce Millan, along with some of his key people, stuck with the issues they had worked on, gaining support for action from members of all parties in the Scottish Parliament. Jim Kiddie worked to ensure that advocacy was not forgotten. Millan asked the parliamentary draftsmen who prepare bills that come before Parliament to state the principles of the new law in its opening clauses. When they said that was never done he pressed them to get on and do it. And they did. (Easier for a former Secretary of State!)

The bill was a complex one. So parts of it – including its clauses on advocacy – were not ready when it was introduced into the Scottish Parliament. These came later and were at once opposed from four quarters. The Nurses' Royal College said that nurses are already their patients' advocates and no other is needed. The Citizens' Advice Bureaux said advocacy is a great idea and they should be paid to provide it. The Convention of Scottish Local Authorities (COSLA) – the 'trade union' of Scottish local government – said money for such a service should be paid to local authorities, but on terms that would leave them free to spend it as they saw fit. And the Scottish Faculty of Advocates – the lawyers' trade union – said no one was entitled to call themselves an advocate except a lawyer.

Those who set up new services never enter a virgin land. They always find that the territory in which they will have to work has already been occupied by other tribes who will try to fight off intruders. Parliaments do not set up new services; they give people powers, resources and a general direction about the things they should try to achieve. These people then have to make what they can of the licence they have been given to act. The outcome will depend partly on the recognition they secure and the settlements they negotiate with neighbouring professions and institutions. And that takes years to work out. The letter from a senior psychiatrist reprinted in the Introduction to this book shows that advocacy still has some way to go before it is generally accepted.

Parliament and the Executive pressed on undeterred. The idea of advocacy attracted broadly based support – from Conservatives who felt the citizen should be defended against the state; from Nationalists who were pleased to see Scotland going its own way and giving a lead to other countries; and from Liberals and Socialists who wanted to help society's underdogs.

The Mental Health (Care and Treatment) (Scotland) Act, as it eventually became, was passed in 2003 and came into force in October 2005. It called for a free advocacy service that would be available to anyone with a mental disorder who wanted it – a local service provided by voluntary bodies that would not be permitted to do anything else but advocacy. This service would be paid for by local authorities through their social work departments and by the National Health Service, with additional money provided, through each of them, by Scotland's central government. Although intended to help people with mental disorders, the service would be launched in an open-ended way that would enable the agencies providing it to extend their help to anyone they chose – provided they could find the money to pay for that. Hector Mackenzie's challenge is still alive.

In conclusion

This is one of several reforms introduced by Scotland's Parliament that show both a belief in the state and its public service professions, and a robust capacity to challenge established authorities. The Land Reform (Scotland) Act of 2003 is another – giving local communities that register an interest in the land and buildings among which they live the right to acquire them if they are ever put on the market. So is the organisation of the Parliament itself, which has a Petitions Committee that hears petitions from the public, meets their representatives and passes their petitions on to other relevant committees if that seems appropriate. This robustly democratic spirit is part of the culture and tradition of Scottish people – going back to Robert Burns and beyond. It is as deeply rooted in the experience of crofting communities of the Highlands and islands as in the trade unions of red Clydeside. The opening of the new Parliament was celebrated with a great rendering of Burns' most famous song, deriding the pomposity of power, and ending:

> For a' that, an' a'that,
> It's coming yet for a' that,
> That man to man the world o'er
> Shall brithers be for a' that.

But the work that will eventually shape this country's advocacy service is still only beginning. These are some of the questions it will have to answer.

- Will advocates 'broaden' or 'deepen' the service they provide? Will they help people with a growing range of needs to deal with a growing range of authorities? Or will they do more and do better for those with mental disorders – the people for whom their service was first set up? Can they do both?
- Will different kinds of advocacy develop – 'peer advocacy', 'citizen advocacy' and so on – with growing support from public funds? Or will the pattern developing under the Scottish Mental Health Act become the dominant model?

- Will advocates maintain their focus on individual clients and the specific problems on which they seek help – doing a short-term, one-off job for each of them, and perhaps strengthening the 'customer' power of their clients? Or will they do much of their work with groups, maintaining long-term contact with their members and fostering a collective 'citizen' relationship to public services?
- Will advocacy help to reverse the tendency – well known in the health services – for the neediest and frailest people to get the poorest services? Or will it reinforce this pattern?
- Will advocates maintain their independence, despite their reliance on public funds? How far will they – how far *can* they – become a campaigning force, confronting public services that fail and challenging them to improve?
- Will their initial reliance on unpaid volunteer advocates be maintained? Or will they become an increasingly 'professional' service – in the sense that they rely increasingly on paid staff?
- What part will service users themselves play in providing advocacy, through voluntary agencies they work for, or in less formal groups of their own?
- How will advocates monitor and audit their own work? Who will make that evaluation? Will advocates or the agencies in which they work have to be formally qualified and accredited to do their job?

These are some of the questions we shall explore in the rest of this book.

THREE

What advocates do:
their main clients

Introduction

In this chapter we describe what advocates do and discuss what we can learn from their experience. This and the next two chapters are the 'engine room' at the heart of our book, showing the work that has been launched as a result of the reforms traced in previous chapters and posing questions to be discussed in those that follow.

Advocates – paid staff and a few volunteers – brought the cases we describe to small meetings where they discussed them with their colleagues. With one or two exceptions these advocates all worked for the same Scottish voluntary agency. Each agency has its unique character, depending on its origins, the people who now work for it and the needs of those whom they serve. So none of them is typical of the whole network. But we are confident that the people working for other agencies of this sort will be familiar with the kinds of stories we tell and the dilemmas they pose.

Advocates choosing cases to present at these meetings were asked to bear in mind the readers for whom we are writing – particularly people who may want to become advocates, those who may have to deal with advocates in the course of other work and others preparing to enter these fields. That meant the cases presented should be real, not imaginary. They should be cases that pose interesting questions – questions that advocates find helpful to discuss with their colleagues. We were not trying to produce a typical cross-section of our work. Some of the cases have successful outcomes, but we did not want to present a succession of 'George and Dragon' stories – cases in which gallant advocates rescue fair maidens from dragon consultants, social workers and hostel wardens. The chapter is neither a research report nor an advertisement for advocacy. We hope it offers realistic, interesting education.

It was the responsibility of each advocate to camouflage their cases with small changes in the story – sufficient to make them difficult to identify but not so great that essential features of the story would be lost or distorted. That is why we have not attached the names of advocates or their clients to individual cases and why we do not name the agencies, hospitals or local authorities involved. Wherever possible, the clients involved were consulted and gave their permission for their story to be included in our book.

People tend to seek the help of an advocate when things go wrong and they feel they have suffered from incompetence, neglect or injustice. That means the glimpse of our health and social services offered by these stories is not typical of the work they do. They usually do better than this. We invited the main local authorities appearing in these stories to read and comment on this chapter and the next one, and we have incorporated or responded to some of the points they made.

Terminology

Before we could start writing we had to decide what words we should use to describe the people advocates try to help. 'Partners', 'users', 'service users', 'customers' and 'clients' are all to be found in other books. 'Partner', we believe, is intended to stress the equality and mutual respect that should be found in the relationship. It may also be intended to distinguish it from relationships with social workers and doctors: professions sometimes required by society to wield power – to confine people in a hospital, to report on them to a court or to take their children from them. 'User', 'service user' and 'customer' identify only one aspect of a person's status. We are all of us users and customers of every kind of service. All of these are rather vague terms and none of them implies any particular duty to be performed by the advocate. 'User' can have a slightly contemptuous undertone. 'Customers' may be expected – and feel entitled – to be as demanding and manipulative as they choose. And advocates who ring up a social worker to say, "I am advocating on behalf of my partner" will have some explaining to do before they can be sure they are on the same wavelength.

We have chosen 'client' as our preferred word because it implies that advocates have duties to the people they try to help. It is professional or businesslike, suggesting their relationship is intended to resolve specific problems and then to come to an end unless renewed to tackle a new problem. And if we learn from the example of lawyers, architects, engineers and accountants – who all adopted the word 'client' for the people they work for long before there were any social workers about – there should be no suggestion of subordination or unequal power. When we want to focus on particular features of a client's status or needs we may also call them 'patients', 'pupils' — or indeed 'service users'. But mostly we will talk about 'clients'.

When distinguishing people according to their needs and condition, we have tried to call them whatever they would like to be called. But there is a good deal of dispute about that. Some people who are ill *want* to be called 'patients' and to claim the rights that patients should be entitled to. Others with an apparently similar condition reject the idea that they are ill at all. They have an identity that may be marked by unusual mental experiences — but that's what they *are*. And they deserve as much respect for that as anyone else. We have generally used the phrases 'people with mental illnesses', or sometimes 'mental health difficulties', well aware that we will not satisfy everyone with either formula. Throughout the book we have used the phrase 'people with learning disabilities' where some would have used 'learning difficulties' to describe those with an intellectual impairment. The term 'difficulties' covers a broader range of conditions and is often used by teachers to describe young people with no intellectual impairment who find it very hard to fit into a normal class.

The fundamental problem posed by this discussion is not about the words. It's about public attitudes to the people involved. While many still feel hostile, fearful or contemptuous towards the people we are talking about, every word or phrase chosen to describe them will eventually become sullied and rejected. Until public attitudes become more respectful, friendly and accepting, every word we use is likely to become politically incorrect before long.

In this chapter we introduce the main groups of clients a Scottish advocacy agency will be trying to help. They are people who have mental health difficulties, people with learning disabilities, frail older people and a few others who will not appear on the lists of all agencies. All these cases concern individual clients. They are usually dealt with over a fairly short period and then closed. Advocacy for groups of people, which usually continues for longer periods, also plays an important part in the work we will be describing. It is so important that we postpone discussion of it until Chapter Five, which will be wholly devoted to it.

In the next chapter we deal with more difficult problems and dilemmas: what to do about unlovable clients, and clients whose aspirations seem quite bizarre, for example; what to do when the wishes of our client seem to conflict with those of her young daughter; and what to do about people who want to be allowed to die when all around them may be trying to keep them alive.

Our main clients

People with mental health difficulties

Most of the people we advocate for have mental health difficulties. Their stories will usually be presented by their advocates, but it seemed fitting to start with a case written for us by a client. We are grateful to him for telling us his story.

When reading or hearing such a story the advocate's job is to listen with respect to their client's experience and to accept it as their 'reality', not to analyse, diagnose or make judgements. (It's the job of other people to do those things.) That is not easy, and it's particularly difficult for those most highly trained to work with people who have mental health difficulties.

This is what one of our clients said.

Hi! I am Joe. I am the eldest of a family of three brothers. We grew up in rural Scotland. As a youngster I had many dreams and ambitions just like anyone else. When I was in my late teens a close bereavement shattered my world and my family's. I found I was coping and trying to be strong for others, but was unaware of the feelings and emotions being stored deep within me.

In my late twenties I was admitted to a psychiatric hospital and was diagnosed with manic depression. This was very concerning to hear but I was given little information about it and about how it would affect me. I spent six months in hospital. It was frightening and I was not sure what was happening to me. After leaving hospital I realised the diagnosis I had been given was now a label and I noticed I was treated differently from others. I felt I was pushed and shoved and made to fit into a pigeonhole. I remained well for five years. Then I was made redundant and became unwell again.

These are some of the stories I have to tell. They explain what advocacy has meant to me.

On one occasion I required a hospital admission on a general ward – not a mental ward. Whilst in the care of professionals I felt depressed and they decided I needed extra medication. I explained the reasons why I did not want this medication due to the side effects it had created for me in the past. Despite the concerns I raised I later became aware I had been given this medication without my consent. I felt upset, annoyed and became rather angry when asked to take the medicine again. Due to this I was again labelled and reported as being aggressive. A transfer was arranged for me to another hospital. I was told where I was going and I explained this was not the usual hospital I was admitted to where the staff know me. I should explain that I am a big man and hospital staff sometimes get frightened of me when I am upset.

It was a long journey and on the way the ambulance stopped and it was agreed that I would be taken to the hospital I wanted to go to. This meant another three hours in an ambulance. When I arrived at the hospital I felt very poorly treated. I felt this episode of illness was brought on by poor treatment and lack of understanding in the general hospital I had been in.

It was then I became aware of the advocacy service through other patients and leaflets. I contacted an advocate and she quickly met with me. I felt I was listened to and understood. I was given assistance, information and felt respected about the complaints I was making. Advocacy helped me to send letters to the Health Board and raise a complaint. Some time later I received a letter from the Health Board addressing some of the issues I had raised. I did not get anyone to take responsibility for what had happened, but I felt empowered by the fact I had received answers and an apology. I feel the use of advocacy here was incredibly helpful to me as I don't feel that if I had raised these things with a member of the nursing staff I would have got the help and information to decide if I wished to raise a formal complaint. By making my voice heard on this occasion I was respected and treated as other people would be. That can be difficult when you feel you are labelled.

On another occasion whilst in hospital on the second night of admission I was put under a short-term detention certificate. I felt this was unnecessary and the treatment I received was too intrusive. I was removed from the open ward to a more secure unit within the hospital. I believe that if more nursing care had been available to me then I would have been helped more, or medical staff might have noticed my needs were changing so I needed additional care and treatment. Whilst on the more secure unit I felt very alone, sad, worried and confused about the section I was held under. I felt worried as my freedom had now been removed.

When the advocacy staff were on the ward I felt I had someone to talk to in a confidential manner and I knew my concerns were being listened to. They explained clearly what the short-term detention meant and the rights I had under the new Mental Health Care and Treatment Act of 2003. I was given independent information and was able through discussion with an advocate and information leaflets to make a decision to appeal. The advocate was able to access private space on the ward and assist me to make telephone calls to get legal advice so I could apply to the tribunal service to have the section revoked.

I feel the staff would not have had the time and information to have spent with me when I needed to be heard. I also feel that nurses at times will close ranks in line with the psychiatrists' decisions and won't hear what you are saying. Or they can tell you reasons that you need to be in hospital and it just feels pointless trying to explain your position to them. I was fortunate that I did not need to go to a tribunal as the detention was lifted and I was transferred back to an open ward.

The transfer was delayed due to lack of beds on the open ward so I had to remain on a locked ward for five days longer than was necessary. But my advocate was able to negotiate that I had access to the hospital grounds and activities off the ward. If I had not had help from the advocacy service I may have spent longer on that ward and would not have had the information to know about my right to appeal.

Through having the experience of using advocacy I feel reassured to know that if I become unwell again and require hospital admission I will be able to contact them if I need to.

The advocate who has been most recently working with Joe felt it might be helpful for her to write a brief account of her own experience and feelings to stand alongside his. This is what she said.

"I am the middle sister of three. We lived in rural Scotland in a family that was rooted in the Labour movement where there was always talk of politics and the social injustices which had to be challenged. As a young girl I wanted to be a nurse, and at 16 I took up a position as a nursing assistant in a psychiatric hospital where I worked for two and a half years. I then decided to see the world and set off on my travels. For the next 12 years I worked in care homes and did community outreach work, often for people with mental disorders. I really enjoyed working with individuals coming from long-term stay in hospitals or care homes and helping them to reintegrate within the wider community. I have always been passionate about people's rights, and helping to ensure they are respected for who they are. This sometimes brought me into conflict with my bosses in care services and I had to learn how to stand up to them on behalf of my staff and the people we were caring for. I saw a job as an advocacy worker advertised and felt it would enable me to make a difference to the lives of hospital patients. My colleagues encouraged me – saying I had the right skills to be an excellent advocate.

"I was really pleased when I was appointed to the post, but it was often very hard to achieve what our clients were asking for, and many of the professionals within the hospital resisted the whole idea of advocacy. I persevered, with good support from my line manager, and now see our service becoming more accepted. Most of the professionals are coming to understand the advocate's role and to recognise the huge benefit we can bring to people's lives.

"I have found in my time as an advocate that I have made an impact on people's lives by listening to them; finding ways of valuing, respecting and enabling them; and by showing commitment in what I do. I often have to be a voice for people who feel they can't ask the questions or challenge the situations and systems in which they find themselves. I take pride in what I do. But you have to have a strong backbone to stand up to those who try to make you feel an unworthy and rather interfering person."

Discussion

Joe's story is that of a man who experiences recurring breakdowns. Early bereavement, the economic insecurity which may at any time lose him his job and unsympathetic treatment from staff who are sometimes afraid of him – all of these, he believes, play a part in his vulnerability. When he is ill, even this obviously articulate man feels it is hard to get people to listen and respond to him because he has been 'labelled' as a 'manic depressive' and an 'aggressive patient'.

Advocacy came to his rescue, not by transforming his mental health or his treatment – the improvements achieved in his circumstances were quite modest – but by listening to him, taking him seriously and treating him with respect. It is this, he feels, that makes advocates different from the people he calls 'staff'.

To achieve that, advocates have to be independent of the services among which they work. They also have to *be* there – right in the ward – and arrive promptly at his bedside when asked. The help that Joe gets is never imposed on him. It always comes at his request. So, by supporting and advising him as he objects or appeals against treatment and finally gets a courteous apology from the authorities, they give him a great sense of achievement. He did it for himself. Professionals who refuse to deal with advocates or take them seriously are rejecting and humiliating their patients. Advocates don't get involved unless their clients exercise their legal right to ask for their help.

Advocacy of this kind does not replace legal advice and representation. Indeed, it helps Joe to get the help of lawyers when he needs that.

The presence of advocates in the hospital helps to reassure him that he is a normal human being and entitled to be treated like one. It also assures him that, if he has another breakdown, he will find people on the ward who will do their best to help him. All of which has therapeutic value.

Joe's present advocate is a young woman who has not long been in the job; which is a good starting point for a chapter written for people who may want to take up this kind of work. She has a passionate commitment to people with mental health problems, whom she regards as fellow human beings, deserving respect equal to that due to every citizen. Her motivation for that commitment comes partly from family traditions of trade unionism and the labour movement – one of many traditions that have fed their influence into the broader stream of advocacy. (Others include a charitable Christian love for humanity and the tradition of radical, public service lawyers – both strong in the US.)

Our advocate is working in an ancient Victorian mental hospital, built of crumbling stone: a place where staff usually stay much longer than the patients – and may become more institutionalised. It provides good, humane care for many of its patients – otherwise Joe would not have tried so hard to get back there when things turned bad for him.

But, like most old hospitals, this is a place where authority is rarely questioned; a place where professional qualifications and the rank orders of status they define wield great power – a forbidding place for a young woman without much in the way of academic qualifications whose job is to challenge professional power on behalf of people who are apt to become classified and labelled in all sorts of demeaning ways. Her capacity to speak for them – no matter how deranged they may seem – to stand up to authorities of various kinds and to cope with the attempts some of them make to put her down owes a lot to the experience of life she gained when working her way around the world, and to the support her colleagues and her manager now give her. But it probably owes most of all to her courage and to her family who nurtured it.

———————————

People appearing before tribunals

Some advocates feel that clients appearing before mental health tribunals may not be those in most urgent need of their help. They would probably not be there unless the health service had given them a good deal of attention. Many of those working in this field would argue that the greatest needs for advocacy are found among people, unknown to the professionals, who have received no treatment at all.

But patients brought before a tribunal are in dispute with the mighty authority of the National Health Service about questions that may be of dire importance to them. They may find themselves locked up in a hospital indefinitely – subject to regular reviews of their cases (after six months; then once a year). There, or out in the community, they may be compelled to accept treatments which they feel to be painful, degrading – even terrifying. There are also patients due to be discharged from hospital who bitterly resist that because they feel safer where they are.

Patients prepared – as the great majority are – to accept their doctors' advice do not appear before tribunals. About 1,300 patients in Scotland are compelled to live in hospital. That is just over one in ten of those in hospital with mental disorders of any kind. So nearly nine out of ten are voluntary patients who might be thought to be free to leave if they wish. In fact, there is no clear distinction between voluntary patients and those who are subject to compulsion. Many voluntary patients know well that compulsion will be brought to bear if they refuse treatment or try to leave hospital. They may be baffled by what is happening to them there. They may feel incapable of finding a home for themselves or anyone to care for them if they leave.

It was the situation of the small minority in dispute with their doctors – and the inadequacy of sheriffs' courts as the main instrument for settling these disputes – that prompted first the Millan Committee and then the Scottish Parliament to call for the creation of a new system of tribunals, and an advocacy service that would help people appearing before them. It would be an exaggeration to say that the reputation of the service will stand or fall by its performance in the tribunals. But if it clearly fails clients going through the tribunals, the value and future of the service will certainly be in question.

(Strictly speaking, the people who make these decisions are described as a 'panel'. Together, all the panels in Scotland make up 'The Tribunal'. But most people call the panels 'tribunals' and this is the word we will use.)

The legal principles governing the work of those who treat and care for people with mental disorders are shaped day by day in these tribunals. So, although most patients never get near one, and those who do so may not be the people most in need of advocacy, advocates must play an effective part in this central arena of the mental health system.

Advocates have no right to advise a tribunal. It is their clients who have a right to ask an advocate to support or speak for them there. Advocates speaking for patients who have asked them to do this must be heard. Patients also have a right to the help of a solicitor, paid by Legal Aid without any means test, and advocates must help them to find one if that's what they want. It would be improper for them to recommend a particular lawyer, so they present their clients with a list of solicitors to choose from. Some of them are very good at this work; others are not. (Sometimes the list grows a bit shorter if a solicitor puts up a particularly disastrous performance.) Patients do not have to attend the tribunal, but they and those who care for them when they are at home are encouraged to do so.

In case they become incapable of speaking for themselves, patients are invited to make 'advance statements' that specify the kinds of treatment they would want and those they wish to avoid – but, so far, few of them do this. (Every patient hopes to get better, so it is not surprising they are reluctant to plan for a relapse.) They are also entitled to nominate a 'named person' – a close relative perhaps, a friend or a fellow patient – who can speak for them to the authorities if that's necessary, and many do this. But 'named persons' speak for themselves and their interests may conflict with those of the patient. Patients may want to go home but their relatives may feel they cannot cope with them there.

Most of the cases coming to tribunals deal with long-term orders that will be reviewed after six months and then once a year. But short-term detention orders, lasting only 28 days and renewable for another 28 days, may also be contested before the tribunals.

To compel patients to accept treatment in hospital or out in the community against their will under a long-term Compulsory Treatment Order, tribunals must be satisfied that:

1   The patient has a mental disorder.
2   Medical treatment that will alleviate the symptoms or effects of the disorder is available and will be provided.
3   Without treatment there will be 'significant risk' to the patient's 'health, safety or welfare' and/or to someone else's safety.

4   The patient's capacity to follow the treatment is 'significantly impaired' by the disorder.
5   Compulsion is 'necessary' because the patient cannot be relied on voluntarily to follow the treatment prescribed.

Convincing evidence must be shown for all five of these requirements. This evidence is weighed according to the standards of civil, not criminal, law, as a balance of probabilities. It does not have to convince beyond reasonable doubt. The tribunal also has to follow some more general principles laid down in the Act. The treatment to be offered should be the least restrictive of patients' liberty that is possible.

Efforts should have been made to find out what patients want and their wishes should be respected so far as possible. The aim is to maximise benefits for the patient, not anyone else.

For short-term orders, which are normally intended to provide time for assessment and the planning of treatment, the requirements are slightly less rigorous. It need only be shown that there is likelihood, not a certainty, of a mental disorder.

These rules may seem straightforward enough. But even their first words can be problematic. What exactly *is* a 'mental disorder'? A frightening tendency to harm yourself may seem to your parents and carers a good reason for keeping you safe in hospital, but probably not to a tribunal unless there are other signs of illness. 'Personality disorder' is defined in the Act as a mental disorder, but some psychiatrists would not recognise it as such, or would not be prepared to say there is any treatment for it. Tribunals may accept it, but usually for patients who show other signs of mental health difficulties.

People with learning disabilities are rarely subject to compulsion unless they also have mental health difficulties. Whether that is a good thing is not altogether clear; it may explain why so many of them get locked up in jails.

Alcoholism and drug addiction, by themselves, are not mental disorders, although they may eventually lead to symptoms that would be regarded as a mental illness. They may also have been brought on by mental illness if patients use alcohol or drugs to dull the pain it causes them.

Electro-convulsive therapy, or ECT, is banned unless the patient consents. The only exceptions to that ban are cases in which another psychiatrist gives a second supporting opinion and the central Mental Welfare Commission approves – which hardly ever happens. Neuro-surgery and other invasive treatments require informed consent from the patient coupled with a supporting opinion. Special rules apply in cases where patients cannot consent because they are incapable of reasoning or of speaking for themselves.

This first glimpse of the principles to be followed by tribunals shows there is plenty of scope for argument about them. It also shows how far we have come since the days, less than a century ago, when homosexuals were sometimes classed as 'insane' and unmarried mothers as 'moral imbeciles' – and some of them locked up for the rest of their lives.

Tribunals have great power. Appeals against their decisions can be made only on the grounds that there was an error in law or a 'procedural impropriety', that the tribunal acted 'unreasonably', or their decision was 'unsupported by the facts'. Thus, although they usually try to be courteous and friendly, they have to work in fairly formal ways.

In fact, they operate in all sorts of ways. Some ensure that advocates have plenty of time to prepare for hearings. Others deliver the papers only a few hours before the advocate has to take the floor. Some try to be as helpful as possible. If patients are unable to travel, they sit in premises close to their homes – or even *in* their homes. Others sit only in one place, which may be a forbidding old mental hospital, without a lift to help frail people climb the steep stairs (49 in one case) to the room where they meet. There the walls may be hung with portraits of the very consultants whom patients are trying to escape from. Some rigorously exclude from the panel anyone who might have an interest in the outcome of their decisions. Others employ consultants recently retired from the hospital in which they sit to pass judgements on their former patients and colleagues. Psychiatrists vary too. Some welcome advocacy because it treats their patients with respect and helps them to bring out points the professionals might have missed. Others are outraged when cross-examined by lawyers and lay advocates. Some tribunals ensure that advocates are given a fair hearing after questioning them carefully about their knowledge of their clients. Others are less helpful.

When some of the more disturbing of these problems are reported by advocacy managers to the headquarters of '*The* Tribunal', where the whole system is managed and supervised, their letters may not even be acknowledged. Clearly we have some way to go before the hopes that the Millan Committee had for these tribunals are fully realised.

Some lawyers regret that so few appeals are made against tribunal decisions because a steady flow of appeals would help to clarify interpretations of the law. They believe the complexity of the procedures for getting legal aid for appeals would deter even the mentally fittest people from applying.

The Scottish system is still taking shape and no 'typical' tribunal case can be described. In the great majority the recommendations of psychiatrists are accepted. That can be discouraging for hard-working advocates and their disappointed clients who feel they always lose the argument. But the fact that the doctors are usually thought to have 'got it right' may be partly because they know that advocacy will ensure that injustice and incompetence will be fairly quickly spotted. And clients may be reassured by finding that their advocates listen to them and treat them with respect.

Two examples pose some of the questions that arise in these cases. The first concerns a man we will call Alan. His advocate, who was an experienced mental health nurse before joining this new service, tells his story.

Alan is a 33-year-old gentleman who was referred to our service two years ago when he was in hospital under a 28-day Short Term Detention Order (STDO) under the Mental Health Act of 2003. The Mental Health Officer (MHO) – a social worker who was responsible for his care – was applying for a hospital-based Compulsory Treatment Order (CTO) because she believed he could not be relied on to take his medicine regularly if left in his own home unsupervised. Alan hated being in hospital and was determined to oppose the application at a tribunal. I therefore offered him our list of solicitors who specialise in mental health law and secured legal representation for him.

During my first discussion with him I noted that Alan's STDO was due to expire within the next few days – before the tribunal hearing. This was to be the first of several procedural errors. If the necessary papers were not lodged before 5pm on the 28th day of the order – a Sunday – Alan would become an 'informal' patient at midnight and be free to leave the hospital. I explained to Alan that unless the papers were lodged his 'section', as it is called, would expire on Sunday night.

On Monday morning I went to visit Alan in his ward and found that the papers had not been lodged on time, so he had been 'made informal' and left the hospital. Unfortunately for him, this was not to be the end of the story. His MHO said she would apply for a community-based CTO. So I met with Alan at his home and explained what all this would mean. He again resisted the application and we attended the tribunal together about a week later.

This was the first tribunal I had ever been to, and I was terrified! I had no idea how the system worked, what would be expected of me or how I would be received. And it wasn't even *my* liberty that was in danger! I feel for all my clients who have to go through this process, take great pains to explain to them what to expect, and do my best to put them at their ease. I make sure they understand that it can be distressing to hear yourself being talked about, and encourage them to let me know if they wish to leave the room.

This was a fairly short hearing because the solicitor had not obtained the independent psychiatric report that Alan was entitled to. He asked the panel to make another 28-day order if they thought that was necessary. We then went on to hear the evidence. Everybody present is given an opportunity to state their case, the patient and his advocacy worker usually going last. Alan did really well, and told the tribunal that the order was not needed because he was perfectly willing to comply with his care plan.

Then it was my turn. I had noted that there had been no mention of 'non-compliance' throughout the hearing. My understanding was that there should be a history of non-compliance before a community order is sought. This would then have to be 'the least restrictive alternative', as laid down in the Mental Health Act. I pointed this out to the panel and was shot down in flames. I was told in no uncertain terms that there was indeed a history of non-compliance – which, in my view, was a questionable matter of interpretation. I endeavoured to show that in this case compliance was not a problem – but to no avail. The tribunal granted an interim order. Clearly the chairman thought I had a bit of cheek to suggest they follow the Millan Principles.

The next hearing had to be adjourned, after imposing another interim order, because the MHO who would have to supervise Alan failed to turn up. The third hearing granted a full CTO which would have to be renewed after one year – despite the MHO's failure to produce a report that the tribunal had requested.

Alan did not attend these tribunals because he saw no point in doing so. After that, no further advocacy was required. So I encouraged him to complete an Advance Statement which should guide those treating him if he had another breakdown and was unable to speak for himself, and invited him to get in touch with me if he needed my help in future.

Two years later, Alan phoned to ask if I would support him at another tribunal where he was appealing against the continuation of his CTO. He had already contacted a local solicitor and a date for the hearing had been set.

Alan's solicitor failed to turn up, so I asked the panel to grant an adjournment so that he could find another. The second hearing had to be adjourned because – once again – we did not have an independent psychiatric report. The third hearing was adjourned because the lawyer who was convener of the panel noted a potential problem with the dates in the paperwork. The solicitor who attended on Alan's behalf at this tribunal had never actually met him before the hearing.

The fourth and final time Alan appeared before the tribunal it was confirmed that he had been illegally detained for one year. The legal member of the panel suggested to Alan that he have a word with his solicitor about this. I appreciated that he might be entitled to compensation, or at least an apology. Later, I was present when his solicitor explained to Alan what had happened, but she said nothing about any action he could take.

I got in touch with Alan a few days later to discuss the outcome of the hearing. He decided to lodge a formal complaint which I helped him to draw up. Four months later Alan is well and continues to comply with his care plan on a voluntary basis. He has just received a letter asking him to send a formal application for compensation, which he had already enclosed with his original complaint. It had presumably been lost.

Now, with many, many tribunals under my belt, I have the experience and confidence to appraise this system. Some may argue that the advocacy worker is there merely to speak up for the client, not to challenge the evidence or engage in independent argument. Others would argue that the advocate should try to achieve a favourable outcome for the client, whatever that takes – within reason. The ability to do this is not something that can be learnt from books (sorry David! [meaning the author of this book]).

MHOs are taught court skills to make sure they understand not only the law but also the etiquette of the proceedings and the manner in which they are expected to present themselves. Advocates need similar training, including supervised practical experience of tribunals at work.

Discussion

Little needs to be added to the final comments of Alan's advocate. The first three of his tribunal hearings took place during the first year after the Mental Health Act came into force in October 2005. It is perhaps not surprising that there was a good deal of confusion still around about the workings of the new system, although it should not have been necessary to hold three hearings to reach a decision that would have been made at the first if everyone had done their jobs properly. But a tribunal convener's humiliating treatment of an advocate shows contempt for her client, who may already be finding the proceedings baffling and intimidating. Alan gave up attending these hearings because he could see no point in doing so and that may well have biased the tribunal against him.

Two years later, things should have been going better. But this time it took four hearings to reach a decision. That decision was favourable to Alan, but revealed an injustice to which the authorities have, at the time of writing, made no response.

Clearly there are many factors other than the client's mental health which shape the outcome of tribunal hearings. Patients appearing before them are entitled to the help of a solicitor funded, with no means test, through the Legal Aid scheme. Fees paid under this scheme have been falling in real value for many years. They are currently £47 an hour for solicitors giving only advice and £57 for those speaking for their clients at a tribunal. Some solicitors continue to do an excellent job for their clients: committed, caring and competent. Others do not trouble – or may be unable – to meet their clients before the hearing, and may even fail to turn up when needed.

Mentally frail people often find themselves caught up in the workings of a machine that would seem bewildering and intimidating even to the most confident citizen. The 'welfare state' should do better.

The next client whose case we present – we'll call him Mike – was a withdrawn 'loner' of a man, aged about 60, with a turbulent temper.

> Mike had spent many years in mental hospitals. Shyly at first, and then more frequently, he would come to our advocates' office, asking for help with small things: writing letters, making phone calls, then speaking up at the reviews regularly made of his condition – steadily gaining confidence. (He was capable of writing letters for himself, but they were presented in a large, sprawling script – a few words to a page – and tended to start with some such salutation as "Dear Cunt". So an advocate's help was useful.)

> Eventually Mike said he wanted to leave hospital and live in the community. But at first no suitable housing could be found for him. With help from his advocate, a housing association was persuaded to offer him a place in a care home and invited him to come and see it – in a building that Mike was absolutely enchanted with. Hospital staff were still uncertain about his ability to cope with life in the community, but his appeal went to a tribunal, supported by

the advocate and a good solicitor, and the tribunal found in his favour. Funds for his care had still to be provided by the Social Work Department whose Resource Review Group, allocating a budget for this purpose, met once a week. Eventually, under pressure from Mike's advocate, they accepted that he must be given a place in the queue, but still released no funds.

That left Mike marooned on the 'delayed discharge list' where patients were supposed to wait for no more than six weeks at most. The care home held their offer open but warned that they could not do this for ever. Hospital staff grew increasingly worried about Mike's mental health as he became more frustrated, angry and threatening – writing letters in his usual style to every authority he could think of. His advocate wrote too – to senior social workers in the hospital and the Social Work Department, and then to the Mental Welfare Commission, which oversees the treatment of patients with mental disorders throughout Scotland – all to no avail.

Finally, and reluctantly, eight weeks after the tribunal hearing, Mike's advocate resorted to the 'nuclear option' – emailing a brief account of the case to the local Member of the Scottish Parliament who promptly emailed the Director of Social Work, copying his message back to the advocate. Thirteen minutes later, funds for Mike's place in the care home were provided.

The home, which stands on the coast, looks like a Victorian castle. "I always wanted to live in a castle", said Mike.

Discussion

The client in this case was the hapless victim of a battle over funding that was being waged between the local authority and central government – the locals piling up evidence of unmet needs to support their demands for more money from the centre. The fact that this frail and increasingly unstable older man was on the verge of a renewed breakdown – leading perhaps to an attack on the staff caring for him – made no impact on the protagonists. Hospital staff welcomed and supported the work of the advocate whose patient, resolute pressure eventually gained attention for Mike's needs. Advocacy was being used as a method of mediating in a power struggle between different bureaucracies.

Without someone prepared to stick with him to demand that the different services involved (Health, Social Work, Social Security and Housing) spoke to each other – someone with the sense to know when to bring up the political big guns – people might have got hurt and

Mike might have ended up as a hospital patient or a prison inmate, perhaps for the rest of his life. The responsibilities of an advocate do not end with a tribunal decision, even when it is a favourable one.

_____

People with learning disabilities

This is a story told by Grace – a mature lady with learning disabilities who asked for help from a support worker to tell people about the experiences she had during what she called "My bad old days".

Grace lives in a semi-rural seaside town. She was made redundant when the factory she had for seven years been supported to work in went into receivership. Like others who have been thrown out of work she was devastated. Things got worse when she was told that the only option for her was to return to the adult training centre she had left years before. She tried the Job Centre but couldn't find a job she could do without support.

After three dreary weeks reading magazines and drinking tea in the training centre she decided she'd had enough, put her coat on and walked out. "I missed my workmates and earning a wage", she recalled. "I felt really confused and there was no one to help me."

When Grace got home her support worker called and told her to phone the centre and say she'd be back in the morning. She refused, and got angry with the people who ordered her to do what she knew wasn't right for her. This didn't go down at all well and she was made to feel that she had done something very wrong.

Grace became depressed and more isolated. Her long-term boyfriend, Tom, had some learning disabilities too. But he had a job and had recently moved into his own flat. So she went to see him and shared her worries. They decided they would have to support each other if they were to have any say in their own lives. So they went to 'the powers that be' and told them they'd be moving in together in Tom's flat.

That, people told them, would be "*very difficult*". There were tears, arguments, worries and outright opposition, but very little helpful support and no one to advocate for them. In time, Tom's family came to accept the idea and told staff in the services Tom and Grace would be depending on that they supported the couple's plans. Tom took on an advocacy role within the partnership and eventually they got joint support from a new worker who started to listen to what they were saying.

While Tom went out to work, Grace and their support worker went shopping, tried new recipes and joined a literacy class and a local ladies' group that met on Fridays. Before long she and Tom moved in together and got married. Their support worker helped them to fix up their home.

Ten years on, they are now in a very traditional marriage. Grace is a talented and enthusiastic homemaker. Tom enjoys his home comforts and encourages Grace in her chosen role; and she takes plenty of 'me-time' when Tom is at work, at advocacy meetings, or watching the football.

In recent years Grace and Tom have become volunteers within the advocacy movement. They are effective self-advocates and also peer advocates for other people with learning disabilities whom they come into contact with. They might also be described as citizen advocates, or lifelong supporters, for each other.

Grace ended her story by saying, "I wish I had been able to get an advocate when I had no voice and no one was listening. Things have improved, but there are still more problems and barriers than there are advocates – and this needs to change to give a chance to people like us."

Discussion

This story, even more vividly than Joe's, reminds us that the pain and the difficulties people suffer when they have mental disorders often arise from the combined impact of the disorder and the economic and social conditions they have to cope with. Grace's independence and happiness were destroyed when she lost her job and got no help from her family. A district in which there have been big industrial closures, throwing many people out of work, will need more mental health services and more advocates until the more vulnerable victims of the disaster have been resettled. Later, Grace and Tom could live happy lives because he had a job and they had a house to live in together. We know nothing of Grace's family, but Tom's played an important part at a crucial stage in the story. The couple needed a bit of help from a support worker to get their home together, but after that they became pretty independent.

More than that, they joined various groups and were able to give a good deal of help as advocates for people like themselves. Within a group who have had similar experiences, people with mental disorders can, with a bit of support, do much of their own advocacy. The story reminds us that different kinds of advocacy (peer advocacy, self-advocacy, citizen advocacy, issue-based advocacy – whose exponents sometimes talk as if these were different and competing churches) can very usefully evolve together, supporting each other.

Day centres are clearly one of the settings in which advocates are needed. Otherwise they may become a trap – a comfortable one, perhaps, but not a place that helps people to take risks and find a way back into the mainstream of their society.

This was a story in which a loving relationship between two people with learning disabilities supported them and enhanced their lives. But – as for any of us – such relationships will not always work out so well. This is a question we return to in the next chapter.

_____

People discharged from hospital

When someone has a serious mental breakdown they have often been through a really bad time before they get into hospital. They may have lost their job, their husband or wife, and many of their friends. They may have run up daunting rent or mortgage arrears. After a spell in hospital they come out – partly recovered at least – to find that all these problems are still there. Indeed, they may have grown worse. Their wife has a new partner, their home may have been repossessed, and the neighbours see them as mad and dangerous. It is not surprising that suicides often happen at this time. So advocates need to be alert to help people who are leaving hospital.

Linda, a middle-aged woman with a good job, was admitted to hospital after a serious breakdown in mental health and several unsuccessful suicide attempts. A year later she was discharged, stronger in body and mind but still frail. She had lost her home and her job and was sent to bed-and-breakfast accommodation for homeless people. This was an upstairs room in a pub. The noise below kept her awake at night and she had to be out of the house all day – sitting in cafés and bus shelters in rainy weather.

For complex reasons, Linda had been given no housing benefit and her social security benefits were not yet in place. She was unaware that she was expected to pay for her accommodation. After six exhausting weeks she was rehoused temporarily in a furnished flat for homeless people – heavily burdened by her debt to the pub. The flat was equipped with 'white goods' and furniture for which she had to pay £50 a week in addition to her rent. Because her own furniture had been placed in store while she was in hospital she had no need for these things, but housing officials insisted they were part of the 'homeless package'. She had a social worker who wrote to the Department about this, but with no success – despite the fact that social work and housing are in this county administered by the same department. So Linda fell into steadily increasing arrears.

She was a conscientious person who always gave priority to her rent and council tax, and that left her £1.90 a week for food and everything else. Even to make a phone call about her social security benefits – a call that might never be answered – was impossibly expensive. She had to forage for food in bins and buy things for 10 or 20 pence from local shops disposing of food that had passed its sell-by date.

An advocate became involved and tried to get help for Linda from the housing service. They refused even to consider her financial problems, but offered her a flat in a village that was miles away, which she took in desperation in the hope of reducing her arrears. This was two months after her discharge from hospital.

At this point her social worker moved to another job so no one oversaw her move. When her advocate came to visit her two days later she found the flat had been left in a disgusting mess. There was unfinished plasterwork, a cracked chimneybreast, broken glass on the floor, graffiti on the walls and doors, and dirt everywhere. The response of the housing service, when approached by the advocate, was to give Linda a 'decorating allowance' of £250. But she was neither mentally nor physically strong enough to make effective use of this. She had rent arrears of £1,200, which worried her a great deal. The advocate repeatedly sought help from the Council Arrears Department, which agreed to stop sending demands for payment for two months. After that it expected her to pay.

Linda has fluctuating mental health problems and complex needs of many kinds for which she will require a comprehensive 'care package' offering her good support. Her advocate has written to the council, recording what has happened and pointing out that it has a legal duty to give special consideration to people who have mental health difficulties. At the time of writing, she has received no reply. Neither has any plan been made to give Linda the care and support she needs if she is to lead an independent life in the community.

Discussion

It is difficult to find words that respond adequately to this unfinished story, but a few obvious points should be made.

Hospitals should ensure that support is ready for vulnerable patients before they are discharged into what is reassuringly described as 'the community'. They particularly need to keep an eye on patients who do not have the support of competent local friends and relatives, and patients who are reluctant to ask for help because they lack the confidence to do so – or because they so desperately want to get out of hospital that they don't want to raise questions which might delay that. Advocates working in the hospital should offer their help to such patients and alert their colleagues working in the community to do likewise.

Health, social work, social security and housing services have to keep in close touch if they are to give adequate help to clients with such complex needs. None of them can work effectively if they work alone.

The advocate in this case kept in touch with Linda and may have prevented what could otherwise have been a suicide. But how does one evaluate advocacy in such cases? And what duty does the advocate or her employers have to confront situations in which services fail so disastrously that a lone advocate cannot put things right and letters to service directors are not answered? What should they do? We will return to these questions in Chapter Nine of this book.

Older and frail people

Most of Scotland's advocacy agencies try to help older and frail people as well as people with mental health and learning difficulties. This is a story of two cases of that kind. We will begin with an introduction to the advocate (let's call her Pauline).

Pauline is a volunteer who first heard of advocacy when an application for funds for this work came to an NHS trust that she was then chairing. She was intrigued by this new project and her trust decided to support it. Soon after, she heard that the agency to which they had made a modest first grant would be offering courses to train volunteer advocates and she applied to join the first of these. She found it fascinating and soon became one of the agency's volunteers. Nobody asked if she would have conflicts of interest when acting for patients of her trust.

One evening, when speaking with others from the platform at a meeting called to discuss the future of a local hospital, Pauline watched a frail older woman rise to her feet to ask, with obvious anxiety, a question about the fate of her husband who was due to be moved out of this hospital. The man chairing the meeting tried to kick her question into the long grass by saying they could not deal with individual cases this evening. But Pauline – the trust chair who was now also an advocate – said she would talk with the woman after the meeting, which she did, uncovering a complex tangle of problems.

This woman – Mary we'll call her – knew the hospital was clearing the ward her husband was in. He would be going to a nursing home. Being very frail herself, and unable to pay for taxis, she would only be able to keep in touch with him if he was placed in a home linked to hers by a bus route running from door to door. There was only one that she could reach in this way.

Pauline accompanied Mary to a meeting with two officials to whom they explained her needs. The officials pushed a form across the table with the names of three homes on it and asked Mary to rank these in the order of her preferences. There was only one on the list that she could reach by bus. One was many miles away and two had no bus service that she could use. Pauline, knowing this tactic would enable the officials to send Mary's husband to her least preferred option by saying beds were not available at the other two, said, "But she has only *one* preference: the home where she can visit her husband". Undeterred, the officials told Mary again to state her order of preference. For about 20 times Pauline repeated that her client did not have any 'preferences' – just a need for a bed in the one home she could get to. Eventually the meeting broke up without reaching any decision. Later, Pauline accompanied Mary to two further meetings and eventually Mary's husband was found a bed in the home to which she could travel by bus.

In the months that followed, Pauline sorted out several other things that were very important for Mary: securing disability benefits, arranging bank transfers, representing her at a social security tribunal and so on. She found she had become 'a friend on call' for a frail and lonely lady. Eventually she managed to close this case.

But word of it got about in the nursing home that Mary visited every day and a couple in their early sixties asked Pauline if she would help them too. Roy (let's call him) had contracted asbestosis from many years' work in the shipyards and was already too weak to walk more than a few paces. He and his wife (we'll call her Winifred) knew he would soon be confined to a wheelchair. So they had been delighted to move into a small bungalow – one of two in the project that had been specially designed for wheelchair users. There was a disabled driver's parking bay right outside their front door. The manager of the housing association that had built the project warned them that there was a minor difficulty about getting cars onto the site, but he assured them this would be soon resolved.

It never was. If Roy and Winifred drove in only briefly to deliver their shopping, their landlord promptly sent them threatening letters, upbraiding them for doing this. So, on Roy's increasingly frequent bad days when he was scarcely able to breathe, they were confined to their house. Their whole lives became dominated by this apparently simple parking problem.

The average age of the eight tenants in this group of houses was 81, so Roy and Winifred were not the only ones involved in this tiresome difficulty. They were particularly distressed to see one of their neighbours tottering painfully out to an ambulance and back for regular visits she had to make to a hospital. And, no matter what they said to the management, nothing was done. Getting together with their neighbours, Roy and Winifred got them all to sign an agreement asking Pauline to represent them.

She began to unravel the problem, despite the refusal of management to provide any information about it. She researched three years of planning files on the project, arranged meetings with the landlords, spoke to the Roads Department and the architects of the project, to community representatives, local councillors, the MSP – who all hoped the matter could be resolved by an amended planning application that would permit cars to use the parking spaces already provided. But Pauline discovered there was a problem about the application that was being prepared. It would never be accepted because the sight lines at the entrance to the project were obscured by a few trees in a neighbouring garden whose owner was not prepared to fell them unless compensated for the 'loss of amenity' he would suffer. And the housing association was not allowed to pay for that.

One of the council officials told Pauline that her clients should recognise that "this is as good as it gets. They have lovely new homes and should just accept that they do not have car access. They cannot have everything in life." That was when she resolved that this battle had to be won. She reported weekly to Roy and Winifred, phoning them or dropping in on what they came to call her "tea and toilet stop". When the tenants brought the local press into play, their landlord became more aggressive. He approached the advocacy agency's manager and told him to rein his advocate in. A community representative connected with the landlord made intimidating visits to Roy and Winifred. Pauline became increasingly concerned about their health, but they too were resolved to win this battle.

Eventually a plan Pauline had long been trying to negotiate took shape. Communities Scotland, through which the government funds housing associations, found the money to compensate the neighbour. The trees were then felled, a new planning application was approved, minor building works were completed and a white line was painted on the edge of the highway to prevent cars parking outside the gate. (That took a few months more.) Finally, after two years of arguments, Roy was able to drive his car into the disabled bay at his front door. One more 'tea and toilet stop', celebrated with a cake, brought this case to an end.

Discussion

As we all live longer and have fewer children than our forbears – children who are more likely to move away from home – there will be more frail and isolated people contending with problems like those described here.

These clients would have stood no chance of achieving these ultimately happy outcomes without the help of their advocate. And their advocate would have achieved nothing had she not been resourceful, well informed, capable of dealing with complex issues and hostile officials – and prepared to devote to each case whatever time it needed. That called for difficult decisions because it meant that other clients had to be neglected or kept waiting.

In both cases Pauline, the advocate, developed warm personal friendships for her clients. Without that, she would have found it difficult to stick with them and they would not have been able to trust her sufficiently. Yet she had to be capable of bringing their relationships to a close – unless some new crisis in her clients' lives leads them to phone her again.

Mary's case – the first one – clearly fell within the field the advocacy agency was commissioned to work in. The even more complex second case shows how an effective advocacy service tends to expand the range of needs it tries to meet. ('Mission creep' is the word the military use for this.) The tenants with a parking problem may have fallen on, or slightly beyond, the boundary of the service the agency was commissioned to provide. But it would have been very difficult to refuse to help them.

Once Pauline had started on what must at first have seemed a fairly simple case, she was led into increasingly deep waters, dealing with a growing network of agencies and services. You never can tell what advocacy will lead to.

Many assume that the officials of local voluntary agencies and local government usually do their best to respond helpfully to those who depend on their services. And they probably do – usually. Advocacy tends to be called into play when they do not, and then they can be oppressive, uncaring and pretty ruthless. Advocates should not be surprised or discouraged. This is why their government and parliament set up an advocacy service to speak for the most easily oppressed citizens.

Parents and carers of children with additional educational needs

The agency that provided most of the cases described in these chapters was asked by one of the two local authorities whose people it serves to extend its work by advocating for the parents and carers of children with additional educational needs. Difficult decisions sometimes have to be taken about the education of these children and the authority felt it would be better if their parents had the help of an independent advocate. So they provided extra funds to make that possible. We believe that advocacy is likely to spread in this kind of way, so it will be helpful to discuss a case of this kind.

> Brenda, a 13-year-old schoolgirl, was losing her sight. She had increasingly restricted 'tunnel vision', which meant she could see a pathway only ten degrees wide ahead of her. This made it increasingly dangerous for her to move around the town and she had several accidents on her way to and from school. Her class teacher asked the Education Department to provide a taxi to transport her, but this request was turned down on the grounds that the cost of a daily taxi could not be justified. They offered instead to provide a bus pass, but this was of no help to Brenda. So a social worker for the visually impaired who was helping Brenda asked for the support of an advocate.

The advocate visited Brenda's home with the social worker and agreed with Brenda's mother that he would try to get the Education Department's refusal of funds for a taxi reversed. He discovered that the Social Work Services' Sensory Deprivation Team had made a report on Brenda's needs, which included a 'risk assessment' that strongly supported the request for a taxi, but this had not been sent to the Education Department. He also asked that department for a copy of their 'policy and procedures' for dealing with cases of this kind. Both documents were shown to Brenda's mother and the social worker, and then sent, with their agreement, to the appropriate official in the Education Department who, after further consultations, reversed his decision and provided a taxi to take Brenda to and from school for six months.

The advocate was pleased to find that people in the Social Work and Education Departments dealing with the case took to each other and arranged to cooperate more closely in future. Brenda and her mother were pleased too.

The advocate also informed the family's local councillor about this case and he took it up with some anger, getting an assurance from the Education Department that the taxi would be provided for as long as Brenda's schooling lasted. The advocate completed his work on the case by speaking rather apologetically to the official who had found himself in the firing line and thanking him for responding so helpfully. His goodwill may be needed in future.

Discussion

This sounds like a straightforward case, sensibly handled, with a happy outcome. But it poses some interesting questions.

The advocate's job was to help parents or carers – that is what the local authority is paying for. Brenda and her mother fortunately wanted the same thing. But what if Brenda had wanted to walk to school, despite the dangers involved? (She might have preferred to walk with friends who would guide her; or to practise and prepare for the days when she might have to walk blind.) There are more difficult cases in which the interests of parents and children conflict – cases, perhaps, in which the advocate's sympathies lie with the children. We describe one in the next chapter. In such cases the agency may be able to find another advocate to act for the child, but it is not at the moment funded to do this – so the decision would not be simple.

The advocate doing this work had quickly learnt that 'risk assessments' and formally agreed 'policy and procedures' are documents that have great power within a bureaucracy. Find out what they say and you may be able to use them to help you get the decisions you want. But officials are perfectly capable of reading these things for themselves. Should an advocate be required to draw their attention to them?

Public administration is not quite so simple. An independent advocate was, in effect, being brought in as a 'hired gun' by the social worker to persuade a more senior official in a more powerful department to change his mind. Provided they retain their independence, advocates can work as 'brokers' to help different departments of a bureaucracy negotiate with each other. This fairly common practice may not be the most inspiring use of advocates' time, but so long as it helps their clients it is a necessary part of their work.

People relying on direct payments or individual budgets for the care they need

The same authority that asked us to advocate for parents of children with additional educational needs asked us, soon after, to advocate for people relying on direct payments, or individual budgets, for their care. This method of funding care, which makes clients the selector, employer and paymaster of those who care for them, is a growing pattern. The local authority decides how much they can spend on each case in the light of the clients' needs and financial resources. The clients decide how to use this money. This puts them in the driving seat.

Our advocate is not supposed to plan, organise or pay for the clients' care; only to help them say whatever they want to say to those who run the services they need and anyone else they have to deal with. But that boundary line can be difficult to draw.

> Keith was offered an advocate when the home care supervisor in the Social Work Department who was helping him make arrangements for care through direct payments was warned by her Finance Department that it was not right for her to get so involved in paying his bills. Since someone would have to help him, perhaps an advocate could sort things out?
>
> Keith agreed to give it a try. He is perfectly capable of understanding his finances. But he is virtually bedridden and certainly housebound. He cannot pick up papers, hold them steadily, or write much more than his signature.

He also suffers from the most convulsive stutter imaginable, making him very difficult to understand. And he seems to have no family or friends who can help him.

Working at first with the home care supervisor, who came with him to Keith's home, the advocate got together bank statements and unpaid bills from care agencies and found many to be missing. After about 20 difficult phone calls the bank eventually understood Keith's request for duplicate statements and promised to send them. But none arrived. There were further confused calls to care agencies and copies of unpaid bills were eventually assembled. Keith's advocate helped him by writing cheques for him, getting him to sign them and then posting them for him. This, the advocate feared, was going a good deal too far. Both of them might be compromised. But there is no one else who can do these things for him.

"I regularly have to hunt in various parts of his bedroom and kitchen for the relevant paperwork", wrote the advocate, "and have come to the conclusion that the only foolproof method of keeping things under control is to be at his house every morning to collect letters from the postie at the door; or to have all this mail redirected to someone better equipped to deal with it. I have asked accountants who already handle direct payments for clients what they would charge for this service. The work is simple enough if the papers are kept in proper order, and I think their charges should be modest."

The council could take over this work, but that would put it back in the driving seat and bring Keith's direct payments to an end.

The possibility of giving the work to an accountant is now being explored. Otherwise the advocate will find himself drawn into a permanent role as secretary and personal assistant to Keith. That would go well beyond the job he is supposed to do. He and his agency might even be brought before an employment tribunal by a dissatisfied care worker.

This council had at first been reluctant to use direct payments, but it now pushes for them – sometimes to meet its own needs more than those of its clients. It used to have a contract with an agency that provided help of the kind our advocate is giving to Keith, but this arrangement broke down. Meanwhile the collapse of another voluntary agency providing care for the council led it to switch a lot of its clients to direct payments (DP) as a way of maintaining the service by keeping the agency's staff employed as independent contractors.

As new patterns of social administration evolve, all concerned will have to learn how to work in new ways. An agreed strategy and procedures are needed. The council has a 'DP Strategy Group', which is working on this. The advocacy agency is to meet with them and is preparing examples of cases like this one, which show the kinds of problems that will have to be solved.

Discussion

Direct payments for care were originally invented in Canada in response to demands from parents who had children with learning disabilities. When parents, dissatisfied with the care their children were being given, were assured they would in future be consulted about the service, they said, "We don't want to be consulted. Just give us the money you are prepared to spend and we will make our own arrangements." But the Canadians created a new kind of job for someone they called a 'broker' who would give clients independent, expert advice that would help them to decide the best ways of meeting their needs. (Likewise, you may need a travel agent – someone you trust who is on your side – to find the best deal for you in the hotels and airlines jungle when you go on holiday.) We seem to have got into this system without sufficiently careful thought and planning. In Keith's case, our advocate was being dragged into a broker role that went well beyond the work his agency had been asked to do.

Direct payments can work well for competent people with physical disabilities, and for anyone with a well-organised and loyal family capable of dealing with the mass of paperwork required. But when clients are severely disabled by physical or mental difficulties and have no one to help them they need a lot more than money to provide for their care. Or, rather, some of the money must be spent on close support from an independent and expert personal assistant, concerned only with the client's interests. That person will be a bit like an advocate, but their role goes further and will have to last longer than the kind of advocacy we are writing about.

If we don't take steps to set up a system like this there is a danger that direct payments will create a two-tier system, separating the more fortunate service users on direct payments from the less fortunate who have to rely on whatever service the council or its contractors provide. On the one hand, there will be those who can choose when they go to bed at night and get up in the morning, and who will help them to do that. On the other hand, there will be those who have to take whatever is offered.

This case provides a useful example of an advocacy agency that does not leave its staff wrestling with impossible situations or that simply pulls out, leaving its clients helpless and isolated. The agency is drawing on its experience to work with the local authority to get the service improved.

_____

We have told some painfully harrowing stories in this chapter, but they are fairly typical of the work going on in advocacy agencies all over Scotland. The next chapter also deals with advocacy for individual clients, telling stories that pose dilemmas of various kinds, picked because they may help us to think harder about the principles of advocacy. After that, in Chapter Five, we turn to collective, or group, advocacy.

FOUR

What advocates do: questions and dilemmas

In this chapter we deal with questions that pose dilemmas for advocates – the kinds of dilemmas that it may be helpful to talk over with colleagues. In a book that will, we hope, be read by people preparing to work in this field it is important to present such dilemmas – not just the easy victories. Our discussion of each is designed to help the reader think about the puzzles involved, not to provide authoritative solutions to them. Dilemmas, by definition, do not have clear-cut solutions that everyone will agree about. Meanwhile, readers should bear in mind that the cases discussed here are not a typical cross-section of advocacy work. They are *meant* to be rather difficult, which also means they do not show the welfare state at its best.

People with fantasies and 'mad' ideas

Advocates have to listen with respect to their clients' stories and concerns. They know they are dealing with people who may have a lot of fantasy in their lives. But this is their reality and, even if some of it is fantasy, this may be what keeps them going in bad times. This was recognised by the psychiatrist in the play *Equus* who envied the passion of the boy, his very disturbed patient, who had a love affair with the great horses in the stable where he worked – a love affair that gave to his life a meaning that was lacking in the psychiatrist's own life. But what if fantasy leads in destructive directions – as it did in terrifying fashion in that play – or simply into fruitless and frustrating dead ends?

How about a man who sought an advocate's help because, living on meagre social benefits, he was determined to buy a house in Spain? The advocate will have to decide when a comforting dream about a castle in Spain reaches a point where it becomes necessary to confront his client with reality. Just to collude in a fantasy is not a respectful way to treat people.

Another advocate was asked to help a young man who, though plainly unable to handle a car, was obsessed with the idea of driving a formula one racer, and exhausted everyone around him by mimicking the sound of roaring engines all day. She explained that it would be impossible for him to drive, but – with help from a friend of hers – she could get him to a practice circuit where he could have a ride in a racing car. Later he was taken to a go-karting park where he could actually take the wheel. Now his family report that he's much calmer and more contented.

We don't all have racing driver friends, but the principle is clear and helpful. "How about someone who wants to be an astronaut?" another advocate was asked. "Explain honestly that this will not be possible", she said. "But try to get him to a space exhibition or museum. Listen seriously and take him as far as he can go."

She also said:

> In such cases I try to get people to talk about their priorities in life. To say what are the things they value most of all in their present lives and what they hope for most of all in the future. Then we can talk in practical ways about the good things they already have and how to get a few more in future.

Sometimes it's not clear where fantasy begins and reality ends.

An older couple, retired from senior posts in the public services, sought the help of an advocate. Very tentatively, the wife (let's call her Janet) who had experienced recurring mental health difficulties, told a story about her childhood. She had, at the age of seven, been sent with her older sister to a convent school where the nuns imposed strict rules of discipline and silence. It seemed as if all the girls were expected to enter religious orders. Janet had vivid memories of a monk, clad in white robes, who came regularly to the school, "looking like an angel". She was an outstanding pupil, excelling in all her subjects. Then, when she was about 12, her sister came to her at the end of the school year and said they both had to leave the school. When they got home her sister said they must never say anything about their experiences there. Later her sister disappeared to distant parts of the world. This unexplained 'expulsion', as she called it, has distressed Janet all her life. Her sister is now dead and she wants to know what happened, why were they expelled, who was to blame?

The advocate found, to her surprise, that the school survives and she drafted a simple letter asking for information about these events, which Janet signed and sent to the school. The advocate was left wondering whether the monk had abused either girl. Did Janet or her sister have a baby – or an abortion? Why did Janet's sister disappear overseas? How much of the story was fantasy? But it was a story she had to take very seriously – standing ready to help again if asked to do so.

People who seem well able to advocate for themselves

The Scottish Mental Health Act, which created the service our examples are drawn from was concerned with frail and vulnerable people. The first advocates recruited to the service did not have to worry too much whether their clients really *needed* help. They did their best for anyone who came to their doors. But, as the service expands to serve a growing range of clients dealing with a growing range of services, it will meet more people who, as expert 'customers' of these services, will be seeking an advocate as one more weapon in their well organised campaign for better services for themselves – a campaign that may exclude other people who have greater need but no advocate to help them.

How should advocates respond? Sometimes – perhaps after consulting colleagues – they will refuse to take on cases in which they believe they are being used in this way. But the decision is never an easy one. An advocate, working in an area where there are many people capable of speaking up for themselves, reminded us that: "When we feel ill or frightened, any of us may need support in dealing with the authorities on whom our fate may depend". "Moreover", she added, "I find that even the people perfectly capable of making their needs known may be simply brushed off. They may need some help before they can get anyone to listen to them."

Meanwhile advocates and the professionals who respond to them should both bear in mind that, no matter how convincing the advocacy, responsibility for deciding on priorities for the allocation of resources remains with those who have always borne it. They will do a better job if an advocate helps to ensure that they really understand their clients' and patients' needs and feelings. The capacity of advocates to do that effectively depends partly on the fact that they *don't* have to make difficult decisions about priorities within the public services.

'Unlovable' people

A resolute commitment to clients from advocates who value and respect them and believe in their right to gain a hearing – these are basic essentials for good advocacy. But what if advocates *cannot* respect a client? Or cannot respect their wishes, which is a different problem?

How about the advocate −a volunteer, perhaps, with young children of her own − who is asked to advocate for a child abuser and finds it very difficult even to contemplate doing that? No one should be compelled to advocate for someone for whom they feel anger and disgust. They are unlikely to do a good job, so it would be equally unfair to the client and to the advocate to ask them to try. But another advocate must be found who feels able to help. It would be disgraceful if their agency started selecting morally acceptable clients and excluding those they regarded as unacceptable.

How about the advocate who has no difficulty with the client himself, but who finds the things for which he is seeking an advocate's help are unacceptable? The advocate's response must again be a matter of judgement, often best arrived at after discussion with colleagues.

Clients may want something that is plainly against the law − illicit drugs smuggled into a hospital or prison, for example, or the replacement of a carer or nurse simply because he or she is black. Advocates have to explain that there are laws prohibiting these things, and they are not allowed to break the law. Neither may they endanger anyone − by asking that electrical equipment be installed in dangerous ways, for example. Nor may they tell what they know to be blatant lies on their clients' behalf. That would damage all their clients by destroying the credibility of advocates.

But these distinctions are not all clear cut. When does avoidance of danger become a refusal to allow the client to take normal, clearly understood risks? (How about that go-kart?) When does a passionate and rather biased version of the truth become a blatant lie? Again, advocates have to make judgements about such things.

How about the advocate whose client wants something perfectly lawful, but unacceptable to the advocate concerned − the client seeking an abortion within the proper time limit, or a withdrawal of the treatment recommended by doctors, deliberately bringing his or her life to an end? Some advocates will find it difficult to give of their best to such clients. But, while an advocacy agency should recognise the right of its staff and volunteers to stay out of cases that pose crises of conscience for them, they should also find another advocate who is prepared to help any client with a legal request.

'Heart-sink' clients

This term, originally invented by doctors for some of their patients, describes their feelings when these patients enter the surgery. Advocates, too, occasionally meet 'heart-sink' clients – people, perhaps, who complain about every service they deal with, and will probably end up complaining about their advocates too. This is the story of an advocate working with a client who received direct payments to enable his wife to live more comfortably.

We sometimes have to fight a client's corner, even when we believe this might not be in their best interest, or may indeed be a totally unjustifiable request. To deflect criticism I sometimes have to stress that only by testing the client's arguments to irrefutable destruction can their detrimental – possibly even dangerous – consequences be demonstrated and the ground laid for rational compromise.

I was asked to help this couple do battle over the rebuilding of what most people would have regarded as a lottery winner's dream home. It had been converted for wheelchair use, with every electronic device, a home cinema, a new luxury kitchen, a car port built, and then rebuilt, to take a jumbo-sized motor home, the driveway and garden rebuilt … and so on.

But still my clients were dissatisfied. By the time I came in, every professional – social workers, housing managers, architects, contractors, surveyors; everyone except one occupational therapist – was refusing to speak to them. They cited a long list of what they believed to be outrageously frivolous complaints made by these clients – and, indeed, the clients handed me such a list.

Having built and renovated a few houses in my time, I felt I was reasonably qualified to make some tactful suggestions that might lead to a compromise. I explained, for example, what planning and building control regulations would and would not permit; why the architect's warning that the alterations they were demanding would bring the roof down over their heads had to be taken seriously; why changes they demanded for electronic equipment would be dangerous, and would deprive them of manufacturer's guarantees and insurance cover – and so on.

I was rewarded with a blank and pitying stare, and admonished never to accept the word of 'so-called experts'. I had not only failed them. I had become one of the enemy. (As a consolation, I had learnt a lot about aspects of building regulations, which will come in useful in my upcoming loft conversion.)

Discussion

As we saw in our Introduction, there are even some psychiatrists who do not yet understand that the duty of advocates is to help their clients say what they want, not to decide what would be in their best interests. So it is not surprising if architects and surveyors also have some difficulty in grasping this. The client's wishes do not have to be shouted at those who seem to be obstructive. It is usually better to convey them – as this advocate tried to do – in ways that may lead to an agreement that will give the client as good a deal as possible.

This principle has all sorts of practical implications. It means, for example, that advocates cannot get professional indemnity insurance that would cover them against giving bad advice. We tried, but had to explain that we don't *give* 'advice'; and we may not believe that what we are asking for is in our clients' best interests. The advocate in this case was doing his best to follow these principles.

One family: two advocates

In the previous chapter we described a case of a girl losing her sight whose interests might have conflicted with those of her parents. Every experienced advocate has met this problem. In one of our cases it quickly became clear that two members of the same family might have conflicting needs and each should therefore be entitled to an advocate of their own. The various agencies they would be depending on might also have conflicting obligations.

A community psychiatric nurse asked an advocate to help Jean who was a mother with mental health difficulties living on her own. Her son, Andrew, aged 16, sometimes came home to be with her. He had attention deficit disorder which made him very stressful to share a home with, but for most of the time he was in a residential special school some distance away.

On the advocate's first visit, Jean, who was a talkative, articulate woman, explained that she wanted to move away and live on her own. She was entitled to do this and believed that, with an appropriate care package, Andrew would cope perfectly well in his school.

The advocate returned to talk with mother and son when Andrew came home. He said he was content with his mother's plans. He knew she was unhappy and he wanted to make things better for her. But he had decided to leave his school because he had turned 16 and was therefore entitled to go. Throughout this discussion, which was led by Jean, he constantly looked to her for approval of all that he said.

The advocate explained her role and suggested that Andrew might benefit from having an advocate of his own. There would be a number of issues and services he would be concerned with for which he might need independent advice. He was keen on that. So the advocate said that, with his consent, she would ask a good volunteer advocate working with her to help him.

It was a complex situation. The advocate was concerned about: (1) Jean's mental health and her capacity for making decisions; (2) Andrew's ability to understand the whole situation; (3) the relationship between mother and son; and (4) the possibility that Andrew might be entitled, under the law, to vulnerable adult status which could be helpful to him.

She brought John, a volunteer advocate, to the next meeting with Jean and Andrew. The atmosphere was strained and the advocates suggested that they meet with Andrew on his own at some other place. That meeting went much better and he was much more at ease.

Because Jean was desperate to move, the Social Work Department arranged a multi-agency meeting for them both. This went on a long time and ended in stalemate because Social Work could not provide care packages for Jean and Andrew within the time scale she felt she could tolerate. They would have to make a full assessment of Andrew's needs before making decisions. They asked him if he would return, for the time being, to his school, but he flatly refused. It was eventually agreed that they would provide more social support for him in order to give his mother some respite. She spoke up confidently for herself at this meeting.

After this, the relationship between Andrew and John, his advocate, developed well. When apart from his mother, and knowing that the discussion would be confidential, Andrew could trust John and spoke freely and less aggressively.

At their next meeting, Jean had been given a date for her move to a house that had been found for her. She was still being supported by her advocate and her community psychiatric nurse. The advocate's job at this stage was to explain the procedures Social Work used for assessing people's needs. Jean was not satisfied with the time it was all taking, or with the department in general.

Andrew's assessment was eventually completed and he was found supported accommodation in a flat not far from his home. He visited this flat with John and was delighted with it. His mother moved away shortly afterwards. Andrew moved into his flat and keeps in touch with his mother who visits him fairly regularly.

Although this is an 'issues-based' service which had to close the case at this point, the town in which it took place is a small one and John meets Andrew from time to time, and maintains a friendly social contact with him.

Discussion

Although fairly complex, this case had three important advantages. The first was that both mother and son were recognised as having mental disorders, and each was therefore entitled to the help of an advocate. If Andrew had been only a neglected youngster with (so far) no signs of mental disorder, an agency that offered him an advocate would have been going further than it was entitled to under the terms of its contract with the authorities paying for its work. That would have left his mother's advocate uneasily aware that in doing her best for her client she would perhaps damage the son who was probably more vulnerable and in greater need of help.

The second helpful factor was that the public services involved tried, after due reflection, to treat both clients as generously and helpfully as they could. That does not always happen.

The third helpful factor was that in small communities like this one it can be easier to provide the continuing, informal support that is often needed when advocacy is no longer required.

Conflicts of interest like this are not unusual. They show that the work of a good advocacy service inevitably puts pressures on all concerned to extend advocacy to a growing range of clients.

These conflicts also affect the public services that may become targets of advocacy. The psychiatric nurses, social workers and housing managers all had to decide whether to give priority to the needs of the mother or the son. The capacity of advocates to give whole-hearted support to their clients depends on their acceptance that, no matter how forceful their pleas, responsibility for these decisions still rests where it always did. They may influence decisions by ensuring that the responsible authorities really understand their clients' needs and feelings. But they are not trying to take over these responsibilities. If they did so, that would lead them into conflicts of interest that would ultimately weaken their advocacy.

_____

The hostile or inadequate service

There are cases in which the frustrations felt by clients and their advocates about the refusal of a service to provide what they believe they are entitled to expect – or even to respond to letters and telephone calls – leaves them baffled and angry. We must have some strategies for responding to these situations. It's not fair to go on sending advocates out to face inevitable rejection – a kind of charge of the light brigade.

First we need to find out why things have gone so wrong. Was it lack of resources, a deliberate policy decision to give priority to other clients and services, incompetence, hostility to the client – or to clients of this type? Different causes will suggest different strategies. We devote a whole chapter to this problem at the end of our book.

> One of our clients needed regular kidney dialysis but neither of the new district general hospitals in his part of Scotland had a dialysis machine. So, to get this treatment, he had to go a long distance to another hospital by taxi at a cost not fully covered by the authorities. He decided he would give up the battle to get this treatment and withdraw his request for advocacy, even if that shortened his life. It was just too much hassle. What should we do? Go into battle for him? Respect his wish to be left in peace? Seek the help of other pressure groups better equipped to talk about this particular technology?

We return to these issues in Chapter Nine, where they are dealt with at greater length.

Sexual rights and duties

Before embarking on a discussion of the rights to a fulfilling sex life that our clients may be seeking we should consider a case that reminds us that difficult decisions with tragic consequences may be involved.

> A couple who both had learning disabilities got married and lived happily without any special support. No one seems to have given them any advice about contraception. One day, feeling unwell, the woman went to her doctor and was told that she was well into a pregnancy that was too far advanced

for an abortion to be considered. She and her husband asked the Social Work Department for support because they did not feel able to care for a baby unaided. Their health visitor asked an advocate to help them because she felt things were being taken out of their hands and they were being given no part in the decisions to be made. The advocate tried repeatedly to get advice for them about parenting skills and a psychological assessment of their abilities before the baby was born, but with no success.

The birth of a baby girl proved painfully difficult and was followed by post-natal depression. The couple were given some support during the day, but the mother received no treatment except ineffective anti-depressants – despite appeals for more help from the advocate. After two months the baby was taken from them and placed in foster care on the grounds that she was "not thriving". A social worker said this would be a cheaper and better solution. That may always have been their intention.

The couple were devastated. "Why did they take her now when we love her so much?" was their desperate appeal. The advocate kept in touch, made sure they understood what was going on and got them occasional supervised visits to their daughter. After three years she was "put up for adoption". The advocate managed, through the Children's Panel, to get a "safeguard" preventing this, on the grounds that there was no evidence that the parents had harmed or neglected the child in any way.

Foster care is now continuing with the same foster parents until the girl is 16. Every two months her parents are allowed to spend a day with her. With help from the advocate, they keep a scrapbook with letters and photos to give to their daughter when she is older "so that she knows that we wanted to keep her and loved her very much".

This is a story to bear in mind as we explore advocacy and sexuality.

Sexual behaviour among people with learning disabilities has until recently been a taboo subject, rarely discussed – as if they had no share in what is for most people one of the most important aspects of their lives. As our society has begun to recognise these people as citizens, playing active and accepted parts in the world, so their sexuality too has had to be recognised and respected. But discussion of it is still thick with myths and misunderstandings.

We sought the help of an adviser and advocate who helps people with learning disabilities who have problems of sexual life and health, and who advises and trains others who work in this field. Some of her clients were happy for their stories to be told in this book, but we were unsure if they really understood the implications of that. So she produced instead the following notes which bring together some of the things she has learnt from their experience.

My aim is to support people with learning disabilities in celebrating their sexuality. Many find this a disturbing and emotive subject. Myths about the sex lives and fertility of people with learning disabilities abound. People believe that they:

• do not have sexual feelings like everyone else;
• are more fertile than other people;
• are infertile if they have Down's syndrome;
• are unlikely ever to get married;
• have higher divorce rates than other couples if they do get married;
• are likely to produce children who also have learning disabilities;
• will lose sexual desires if they are sterilised;
• will find that sterilisation will eliminate the problem of heavy periods if they are women.

Every one of these beliefs is untrue.

The history of people with learning disabilities needs to be understood. Many of them have lived until recently in huge institutions – long-stay hospitals where, despite the bleakness of their lives, they had freedom to wander around the grounds, to have sex when and with whom they wanted, to develop loving relationships and to masturbate. But most of these hospitals have closed and those who used to live in them are now in their own homes where people who are paid to look after them visit them. They have lost contact with the friends they lived with for many years. Loving relationships came suddenly to an end and their sex lives were abruptly cut short. Although living in their own homes has many advantages, the emotional losses they have suffered have, for many of them, been devastating. They now face a huge range of problems. These are some of them.

• They want to have a life partner but have no way of meeting anyone who is not paid to come and see them.
• They pick up messages that, for them, sexual pleasure is wrong – out of bounds.
• They may not know how to pleasure themselves and may hurt themselves trying to do so.

• They may want to have children, but may have been sterilised without anyone telling them this was done.

• If they have fertility problems they find it very hard to get access to the services that could help them.

• They may look at other couples and wonder why their own lives are so different.

• They may touch people inappropriately and get in trouble with the police for doing so.

• They may find someone who could be a long-term partner but they are not helped to live together, to marry, to have children or even to spend time alone together. Indeed, they may be discouraged from doing these things.

• They may want a same-sex relationship but are denied opportunities for this because other people's homophobia gets in the way.

• If they find themselves in a marriage which they want to end they are almost forced to stay in it by those around them.

• They may want to have safe sex but do not know where to get condoms or how to use them.

• They may be told to use contraception but are given little choice about the methods to use. It's Depo Provera or nothing. (This is an injection that sterilises a woman for three months – longer, if repeatedly administered. It should not be used without careful discussion. For some people it may be appropriate, but there are medical and religious reasons why it may be inappropriate for others.)

• They have little or no access to appropriate sexual health and information services.

• They are treated like children, whatever their age.

• Decisions are made for them about their lives without consultation or warning.

• They may not even have any choice about their clothes, make-up or other personal things.

• They are very unlikely to get access to any sex toys.

Some of these problems were present in the case described earlier in this chapter of the couple whose baby was taken from them.

These things are gradually changing. People with learning difficulties are now often supported in living full sexual lives. But they may still lack help in dealing with these questions. Getting the information and services they need; finding a partner; negotiating safer sex and contraception; and getting support and counselling about relationships – all these may be difficult for them. They may also ask advocates for help in rediscovering old friends and partners they have lost touch with.

Imposing 'empowerment'?

'Empowerment' is an idea that came, very appropriately, from the race and women's lobbies, via the groups concerned with learning disabilities to the broader field of mental health. There it may be more questionable. The average middle-class person doesn't want to be 'empowered' by the accountant completing his tax return or the solicitor arranging the purchase of his house for him. He wants these professionals to fix things and let him get on with his own work. *Groups* of people we work with who have experience of using the mental health services probably want to be 'empowered' – at least a bit. But I suspect a lot of our individual clients are less certain about that. We do not have a case to offer that illustrates this dilemma. But we should always ask, do people *want* to be 'empowered'? When is the idea appropriate? Do we sometimes manipulate them rather unwillingly into empowerment? Is there anything wrong with doing things *for* people if that is what they would prefer?

Cases that cannot be closed

The publicly funded Scottish advocacy service is designed to help people sort out one-off problems. In theory, the case is then closed unless and until the client comes back to ask for help with another problem. But some people, and some families, are so frail – and so neglected by other services – that responsible advocates may have great difficulty in drawing the work they do for them to an end. Here is a case of that kind.

> Karen is a young single mother with a three-year-old daughter. She was referred to advocacy because she had moved from a big city to a smaller town and the comprehensive package of care to be transferred with her had not been properly organised. She has a desperate history of abuse, first in her childhood, then from a partner. Leaving him, she took up with a 'boyfriend' who encouraged her to work as a prostitute. Heavily addicted to heroin, and suffering all sorts of mental and physical illnesses, she came to the attention of the authorities when she became pregnant – her boyfriend still insisting she continue with her 'work'. Karen managed to come off drugs and get rid of him about the time her advocate came on the scene.
>
> So she was a tough young woman. She had been given a diagnosis of 'personality disorder', which she disputed. This made it difficult to get her a psychiatric assessment, despite the mental distress her advocate noted every time she

made her weekly visits. Working together, the advocate and Karen's social worker eventually managed to get a psychiatrist and a community psychiatric nurse to visit her at home. Unfortunately she appears to have held them hostage there and they now refuse to have anything more to do with her.

The advocate resolved that she must now close the case – Karen's problems fell increasingly outside the field she was supposed to deal with. But within a few weeks she was back on the phone seeking help to prevent her child from being taken from her. So, because she had spent so much time with her and there was no one else likely to help, the advocate reluctantly came again to her aid and is still wondering whether she will ever be able to abandon her. Over a period of several years she has dealt with some 20 different problems for Karen, ranging from debts and rent arrears to disputes with neighbours, from illnesses of many kinds to getting legal aid and help from Women's Aid – and much else. "What she really needs", said the advocate, "is a competent pal".

The mental health worker who is Karen's 'key worker' is still unclear what exactly the advocate's role is. "I think she believes me to be an additional support worker", the advocate said, which in a way she is. But should she have allowed that to happen? Should Karen's key worker have given this service?

Discussion

This is a case where a competent 'citizen advocate' is plainly needed – a volunteer who sticks by someone for life, giving them the kind of support they might get from a loyal friend. But the people who most need this sort of help are not the easiest people to befriend. And, anyway, there are no citizen advocates in this area.

This is not the first story we have presented that shows how staff in other services sometimes bring advocates in to help their clients get services they have failed to secure for them. Which is a legitimate tactic. But, once involved, there is no telling where the client's needs may lead. It can be very difficult for advocates to withdraw from their clients' lives. They need the support of colleagues not directly involved in the case if they are to take what may be a very hard decision.

Death wishes

Advocates working with frail older people, as Scotland's often do, will get involved from time to time in the decisions their clients wish to make towards the end of their lives. *How do I get to Switzerland* (where assisted suicide is legally available) and *Can you help me make a living will?* are questions they are familiar with. This is contentious territory, so we must briefly clarify the history underlying such cases.

A hundred years ago, when death approached, the great majority of our people would be lying in their own beds with close relatives nearby. They might be visited occasionally by friends, a nurse or a doctor who could do little more than make the patient as comfortable as possible. Later, their bodies would be laid out and the neighbours would come to pay their last respects. Death was a domestic and a community event, its timing decided by nature.

Today, most of us will die in hospitals or other institutions, surrounded by strangers and tended by people in white coats with the technology to keep us alive for a long time. Death has become – and will increasingly become – a public medical event, its timing decided by doctors.

Patients are increasingly demanding that their voices be heard when that decision is made.

If they want their lives prolonged as far as possible, doctors can do their best for them. But if they seek help to bring their lives to a decent and painless end they run into all sorts of legal and professional obstacles. They have a right to refuse treatment, but they may no longer be able to speak. Doctors are frightened of shortening life without good reason. Morphine, which was Dr Shipman's favourite murder weapon, is now prescribed more sparingly. In the UK, assisting a suicide is a crime, which may get professionals struck off and can lead to a fourteen-year prison sentence.

Middle-class patients with doctors among their close friends and relatives will often get discreet help in drawing their lives to an end. But too many people find themselves hapless victims of pain or humiliating dependence on strangers, watching their loved ones buckle under the burdens they unwillingly lay on them. Meanwhile many more fear this may become their fate.

So it's not surprising that, for years, every survey of the British population has shown that large and growing majorities of our fellow citizens (now about 80 per cent) would support the legalisation of voluntary euthanasia in the kinds of cases most of us would regard as reasonable – subject to the safeguards that more civilised nations like the Netherlands have worked out to protect us from unscrupulous relatives and people like Dr Shipman.

But most politicians who were prepared to introduce family allowances, abolish the death penalty, take us into Europe and into the Iraq disaster – all opposed by most of their people – are not prepared to accept the views of this massive majority. That's probably because well-funded and strident spokesmen of right-to-life groups oppose such a reform, while the dead and dying have no votes.

So, while we await politicians courageous enough to tackle these difficult issues, patients, their loved ones and their doctors have to decide how best to deal with end-of-life decisions. Advocates, unavoidably, are among those who get involved.

It is their duty, we believe, to listen with respect and sympathy to their clients, who may be in great distress, and help them to achieve whatever they want, provided it falls within the law. If they want doctors to prolong their lives to the last possible moment, they are entitled to ask for that. If they want to bring their lives peacefully to an end, they are equally entitled to ask that treatment be withdrawn. But that is as far as advocates can go. Their concern is to support their patients as far as the law permits, not to take sides in the great debate about euthanasia.

Anna, a lady in her nineties, with no relatives except two nephews who were at sea in distant parts of the world, became seriously ill in the care home where she lived and was taken to hospital, where they told her she had not long to live. A friend visiting her there was very distressed about this because she knew Anna wanted to go back to the house where she had previously lived, to accept no life-prolonging treatment and to die there. So she sought the help of an advocate who found that the local authority had a fund to pay for terminal care in such cases. She helped Anna to write a letter expressing her wishes and to sign it, and sent copies of it to her solicitor and her nephews. Anna was moved back to her old home and two carers who knew her well looked after her until she died a few weeks later. The advocate was invited to her funeral.

In another case, the same advocate helped Margaret, a client who was extremely ill but had been repeatedly resuscitated, against her will, at the insistence of relatives and carers. Margaret was barely able to speak but the advocate managed to ascertain her wishes and to write a living will that she was able to sign. This asked that she be allowed to die when her next relapse took place. Meanwhile the advocate arranged a meeting with her relatives to explain her wishes and the living will. "This was very upsetting for all concerned, but it took away responsibility for decisions from them and fulfilled Margaret's wishes. She passed away five weeks later – her wishes complied with." Once again, the advocate was invited to the funeral that followed.

The people we never hear from

Scotland's advocacy service will never reach all who need its help, or even those who need it most. We should bear in mind the 'law of halves' formulated by Julian Tudor Hart. In many countries, whole-population studies – studies, for example, of every patient on a GP's list, or every resident in a care home or a prison – repeatedly show that, for both mental and organic illnesses, only about half of those who have a particular condition are known to any health professional. Of *those*, only half receive any serious treatment and, of those, only half benefit significantly from it.

Thus, in a town with an adult population of 10,000, about 100 (1%) will have schizophrenia. Of those, only about 50 will be known to the health services; about 25 will have had some serious treatment; and perhaps a dozen will have benefited from it. (Even more worryingly, the same proportions apply when studies are made of people living in hospitals, prisons or other institutions where they should all be under professional care.) Advocacy will always tend to focus on the thin, tail end of this sequence, among those known to the professionals and getting some treatment.

Couple the law of halves with the 'inverse care law', which tells us that, unless special steps are taken to break free of it, the individuals and communities with the greatest needs for care always tend to get least, and it is clear that advocacy, by itself, is not going to transform the world. First hospital admission for poorer patients who have schizophrenia comes eight years later, on average, than for richer patients. Advocacy will always tend to focus mainly on those who are getting some treatment and neglect a lot of those who most need it.

That should not deter us from doing the best we can for those who do seek the help of advocates. But we are left with disturbing questions. Should we also be trying to find and help those we never hear about? How do we do that? An example will show the kind of person we are apt to neglect.

An advocate was asked by a social worker to help a man in his forties who was on the brink of being turned out of his aunt's flat and becoming homeless. He had learning disabilities, was depressed and unable to read. But the advocate helped him negotiate his way into a temporary flat for homeless people, which was clean and well furnished. Visiting him two days later, she found him very proud of his new home and asking if he could get his brothers to paint it. This "would give them something to do". Meanwhile, he would like to do some voluntary work. The advocate set up all these hopeful possibilities and asked for a support worker to keep in touch with him. But on her next visit he was having trouble with the washing machine, vacuum cleaner and central heating. Soon after, he disappeared and has not been seen again.

Discussion

This was a man on the fringe of a much larger group of homeless and semi-homeless people, some of them sheltering in skips and under bridges. One of his brothers has since sought the help of advocates. If we can help one or two of them successfully, others turn up as the news spreads. Traveller families in rural areas show a similar pattern. When one received useful support from an advocate others emerged to ask for help. But soon they drifted away again. There are many more people in need of advocacy whom we never hear from.

In conclusion

This chapter, we warned, deals with problems and dilemmas. Thus many of the cases we have presented are difficult – some of them harrowing. Much of the work of an advocate is more straightforward. Nevertheless, every experienced advocate will be familiar with cases of this kind.

Together they pose many difficult questions, some of which we will consider later in this book. Should we accept a client's fantasies? When should we challenge them? How much time should we devote to people who appear well able to advocate for themselves? How should we respond to 'unlovable' clients and those we have called 'heart-sink' clients? How should an advocacy agency contend with inadequate or uncaring services? Should it get into campaigning roles? How can it best help people with learning disabilities who are looking for sexual partners? What should it do about cases that cannot responsibly be closed? How best can we support people who ask for help in making decisions about the closing stages of their lives? What should we do to reach the people who have never heard of advocacy, or of half the services it might help them get access to?

These are hard questions, calling for difficult judgements by advocates. They pose further questions about recruitment, training and management, and the support that advocates need to cope with the pressures of their work. This is a new profession, formulating ideas and principles 'on the hoof', creating and developing a tradition day by day. Its members need opportunities to reflect on what they do and where they are heading.

The practice and traditions of advocacy will not take a robust and reliable form unless they are supported by convincing procedures for evaluating the work and reporting on the performance of those who do it. Evaluation is a subject sufficiently important to call for a whole chapter to be devoted to it.

Before we go further in exploring these questions we should look at the work that advocates do with groups of their clients. That is the theme of our next chapter.

FIVE

Groups and communities

Introduction

Most of the advocacy funded by the state is always likely to be focused on individuals dealing with one-off problems. But collective advocacy by groups of service users must continue alongside this work.

Individual advocacy can help people cope a bit better with the world they live in. But it never reaches some of those who most need this help. And it may too easily reinforce the assumption – encouraged by much government policy – that each of us has to fight our own corner in the public services market place to get the best deal we can in competition with every other 'customer'. It is only when people who share similar experiences of the public services get together that they can start thinking seriously about changes that may be needed and pressing for action to bring those changes about. As voters and taxpayers speaking for many others whose expertise has been gained from experience of these services, they can in time wield considerable influence. Then things can be improved for everyone – including those who have never met an advocate.

Groups form for all sorts of good reasons – therapeutic, educational, or simply as supportive clubs of friends. This chapter deals with groups that help their members and others like themselves to get the help and treatment they should be entitled to and to bring about improvements in the services they all depend on. While they may do other things too, it is their advocacy we shall focus on, relying on Scottish examples because there is much innovative work of this kind going on here. We describe groups known to us that are doing interesting things, without claiming that these give a comprehensive or typical picture of what is happening in this country.

People in these groups are embedded in various ways in the communities from which their members are drawn. That community may be the staff and patients in a hospital, or just one hospital ward; they may be the people using a day centre, or anyone with mental health or learning difficulties who lives in a particular neighbourhood or city. To bring about change the group will have to influence other people in these communities – doctors, health service managers, politicians and the various 'publics' to which these people respond. So, to understand how groups work, we must also consider their relationships with the wider world.

The Millan Committee, which wrote the great report on which the Mental Health (Care and Treatment) (Scotland) Act of 2003 was based, was very clear about the importance of these groups. They called for a law that would not only provide advocates for individuals who depend on mental health and social care services but also oblige these services to support and listen to groups of service users. The Committee itself had spent a lot of time listening to them and included among its members leading spokesmen of such groups.

This emphasis on the importance of groups and communities forms part of a more fundamental, and very Scottish, conviction that there *is* such a thing as 'society'. We are not only individual 'customers' of our public and voluntary services. We are also citizens, and members of various communities, with duties to our neighbours and the state.

We start by briefly describing the kinds of groups we will be talking about; how they form and what links they have with the communities around them. Then, in the following pages, we give examples of the advocacy in which they get involved. Each of these sections of the chapter will be divided into two parts: the first dealing with groups of people who have mental illnesses – or, as they may prefer to say, mental health difficulties – and the second with groups whose members have learning disabilities.

How groups form

Groups of people with mental illnesses or mental health difficulties

Groups of patients may get together in hospitals, in clinics or day centres. Or they may consist of people with shared concerns scattered all over a town. Professional staff and volunteers may play a leading role in getting a group together and helping it to work; or they may act as supporters of a group in which service users play all the leading roles. Some money will be needed – to pay support staff, rent a room, distribute papers and so on – so there will usually be an agency of the state or a voluntary body somewhere in the background, or sometimes in the foreground.

The group may have been formally elected to represent a larger community of people with similar interests and have a duty to report back to them regularly. Or they may have got going in a much less formal way. The obligations most public authorities have to consult and involve users of their services mean that any group that keeps going for a while will probably be asked to send representatives to sit on planning bodies of various kinds. Thus they have links of varying strength and formality within their society – 'downwards' to a wider community of their supporters and 'upwards' to the authorities on which they depend for the services they need. Their effectiveness depends on keeping both these channels of communication in good working order. Public authorities may be tempted to feel that they have fulfilled their duty to 'consult' if they get a representative from one of these groups to join their advisory committee. Vigorous groups that represent a wider community will not allow themselves to be used in this way.

The needs of their members will vary widely and, because they usually prefer to look hopefully ahead rather than dwell on past illnesses, the clinical character of the group will often be unknown, even to its own members. Indeed, members may reject altogether the idea that they have an illness. They are who they are. If part of their identity and character reflects experiences that others would call an 'illness', that is more a problem for the others than for them. (R.D. Laing and Maxwell Jones would have understood.) Many of them will have bitter memories of being treated with scant respect by staff of the health and social work services, and by colleagues, neighbours and relatives. As their lives move on, taking group members in and out of work, in and out of treatments, the group's membership and dynamics are likely to change continuously. Consistency and coherence may be difficult to maintain, but life will not be dull or uncreative.

Meanwhile there will be other people who feel they need skilled treatment and care, and are happy to describe themselves as 'patients' who are 'ill' – at least for the time being. This is an identity they want to shed, not to deny. Such people also have important contributions to make to the service user movement. Each kind of person and the different kinds of groups they choose to form deserve to be treated with respect. Which is why this chapter – confusingly perhaps – uses both the language of 'illness' and the language of 'health difficulties'.

Groups of people with learning disabilities

We turn next to groups of people with learning disabilities. There are people with complex needs who may be found in both types of group; those with learning disabilities may also have mental illnesses. But groups with learning disabilities generally have a different character. Often they will be based in a day centre, a college, or some other place where their members come on certain days of the week. They may have been elected to represent other users of these services, so – elections working in their usual way – they will probably be among the more articulate and less impaired members of their community.

People who have learning disabilities usually have a lifelong condition, which they learn to manage but cannot escape from. They may have been meeting regularly for many years. Comradeship and laughter grow up between them. Supporting staff will probably turn over faster than group members. Some of these members will also have quite severe physical disabilities. They may be in wheelchairs, may depend on support workers who bring them to meetings and may need help with transport to get them there and back.

Their concerns, when it comes to advocacy, will probably start from the daily routines of their day centre, their college, their transport services or catering arrangements. But they need not end there.

Advocacy

How much can any of these groups achieve? We offer no systematic evaluation – only a glimpse of the activities of a few of them, followed by some reflections on the lessons to be learnt from their experience.

People with mental illnesses or mental health difficulties

Active groups of this kind have quite a long history. HUG – the Highland User Group, based in Inverness – was active well before the Millan Committee began work, as was the Edinburgh Users Forum. Both played important parts in the work of Millan's Committee.

In Edinburgh, along with four projects providing advocacy to help individuals and a user-controlled Law Centre with solicitors who specialise in mental health law, there is the Consultation and Advocacy Promotion Service (CAPS), which helps groups of service users to campaign for better services. The most active of these is the Edinburgh Users Forum (EUF), which meets once a month in a public library and distributes an excellent monthly newsletter. For a while it had a subgroup called KnowUs, which offered training for people working in various public services. There is also the Patients' Council, based in the Edinburgh Royal Infirmary, which holds bi-monthly meetings for patients and former patients of the hospital, and runs a weekly drop-in centre and small working groups. It conveys patients' views to the authorities. Meanwhile the Edinburgh Carers Council provides information meetings for those caring for people with mental disorders and helps them express their views to the authorities. This city has an impressive array of collective advocacy groups concerned with mental health. Reports of the discussions at meetings organised by CAPS are simply but vividly summarised and circulated to anyone interested in them. A recent report from a Midlothian group supported by CAPS listed seven sets of conclusions reached in two, day-long 'have your say' discussions under the following headings:

1   **We need to feel listened to**. For example, "Service providers must … show that service users' comments and suggestions are being taken on board".
2   **Staff attitudes and the way they behave towards us are important.** For example, "There should always be a member of staff on hand and visible for service users to approach".
3   **We need to feel encouraged**. For example, "Make service users aware of the skills they already have and how they can use them in positive ways".
4   **We need to feel confident that services will keep going.** For example, "Make sure there is enough funding and staff cover to continue services and activities, so they are not cancelled".
5   **We need to have a positive experience of using services.** For example, "Space [should be] made available offering some privacy to 'chill out' and/or talk to a member of staff if we need to".
6   **Services must be accessible.** For example, "Referral routes must be kept open, self-referral should be encouraged where possible".
7   **We need to feel involved.** For example, "Service user representative/s should be permitted to attend staff meetings to bring up service user concerns".
    (The language used – "referral routes" and the like – gives clues to the professional experience an Edinburgh group of this kind can bring to the discussion.)

CAPS' paid staff understand very well that it's their job to be a sort of civil service for these people. In the groups they support – the management and executive committees of the Users Forum, for example – only users and former users of mental health services are entitled to vote.

These user groups have a remarkable list of battle honours – things that have been achieved which they believe would not have happened had they not campaigned for them. High on that list is the independent advocacy service for individuals and groups introduced by the 2003 Act.

After 13 years of campaigning that began nine years before this Act came into force, Edinburgh is to set up a Crisis Centre, which is expected to have a help line operating for 24 hours a day, seven days a week. Those referred to it will be accepted at any time and offered one-to-one help, a rest room to 'chill out' in and a bed for the night if they need it. A Crisis Team is also being set up – ready to come to people's homes at any time and provide emergency treatment that has previously been available only in hospitals. CAPS has now been commissioned by Edinburgh Council to review and report on all the day services available in the city for people with mental health difficulties. Professionals – psychiatrists, nurses, social workers and others – also play key parts in setting up these projects. But user groups asserted their needs and made sure their proposals were not forgotten. In doing so they have gained confidence and a sense of empowerment.

More subtly, this movement of independent but related groups is gradually changing the assumptions, strategies and language of the public services working in this field. The innovations they have campaigned for all get people help without them having to go to hospital unless that is really necessary. All start from the assumption that new developments should be planned in close consultation with service users and then evaluated with their help. It has become increasingly accepted that people with difficulties of various kinds should be entitled to decide the words used to describe themselves. Those who used to be described as 'mentally ill' – or worse – are, in these discussions and publications, described as having 'mental health (or mental health and well-being) difficulties'.

People with learning disabilities

We take our examples of group advocacy for people with learning disabilities from two former industrial towns on the other side of Scotland – different and smaller places.

The people using two day centres supported by the same local authority have each elected about eight people to represent them in dealing with the centre's managers and the wider world. Some come in wheelchairs. Some are accompanied by support workers. They meet about once a month with help from an advocate employed by an agency funded by the local authority and the health service. Group members are encouraged to think of themselves as representatives of the people who use their centres, and to bring their ideas to these meetings and report back to them afterwards.

These are some of the things they have achieved. They have protested when let down by the buses that bring some of them to these centres and gained some improvement in the service. They have persuaded the community policeman who sometimes attends their meetings to put parking tickets on cars that are parked in ways that endanger them as they enter and leave their centre. They have secured a camera for the centre, which can be used to record the number plates of badly parked vehicles. They have pressed for, and got, improvements in equipment for the centre's café.

Looking to the world beyond their centre, they have joined with many other people in demonstrations to save a local hospital threatened with closure, drawing and painting the posters they carried on the march. (They have learnt that if you leave a large poster with officials and politicians when you lobby them they will find it harder to file it away and forget it – they might even put it on their office wall.) Some of their members have participated in a delegation taking a petition to the Scottish Parliament, seeking changes in the law dealing with people like themselves. On another occasion, they visited the Parliament, were welcomed by their MSP, introduced to the Minister of Health and shown around the building.

When yet again 'consulted' about proposed changes in public services, they said it was time they did some planning for themselves. With help from advocacy agency staff and a grant from public authorities, they prepared a report with recommendations that are being taken seriously by service planners.

Following from this, some of them were invited to help in training bus crews. What they said was: "Remember some of your passengers cannot run down the street. Give them time to catch your bus." "Some of them will need help when climbing into your bus and stepping out of it." "Some will need help in handling money." "Make sure they sit down safely before you let the clutch in." "Some will not know where to get off unless you shout out the names of the stops."

Another group of people with learning difficulties in this area came recently to a conference of general practice managers, dividing up to talk with them in smaller workshops about their experience of health services. There was lively discussion, a lot of rueful laughter and a massive vote of thanks to them in the feedback forms at the end of the meeting. Since then, they have been invited to do the same things at other conferences.

Activities of these kinds have given greater confidence and competence to people who were previously excluded – even hidden away – from the public life of their town. They have learnt how to conduct elections and meetings, how to address large audiences, and how to paint pictures or stage dramas that get across the things they want to say. Indeed, thanks to the help of a remarkable advocate, they have gained more effective access to the power structures of their society than most citizens will ever have.

By asserting their cheerful and friendly presence on the streets, in the bus queues, the shops, cafés and swimming baths, these groups have helped their towns' citizens to recognise and respect them as members of the community. MPs, MSPs, councillors, journalists, policemen and officials have come to their meetings and gained greater respect for them.

Conclusions

There are many other groups throughout the United Kingdom speaking up for people with mental health and learning disabilities, some of them widely known and operating on a national scale. Most of them focus on the needs of people with particular conditions – schizophrenia, Alzheimer's disease, autism and so on. In this chapter we wanted to learn from the experience of locally based groups of people brought together, not by a particular diagnosis but by shared experiences of public services, to assert their needs and campaign for improvements. What lessons can we learn from them?

First, and most important, it is possible for people advocating for themselves as a group to make an impact on policies that shape the development of services that they and many others depend on.

We all benefit from that. When minorities hitherto excluded from policy debates at last gain a hearing, they do not just demand more and better services for themselves. They bring a perspective to bear that can help us all. Who would not be grateful for bus crews trained by people with learning disabilities? The health service managers who learnt from the same kinds of people how to give better treatment to such patients in their surgeries and clinics will take better care of all of us. The same can be said for people with physical disabilities who have persuaded architects to make their buildings attractive and easy to use for people in wheelchairs, people who cannot reach floor-level electric sockets and people who cannot turn a conventional tap on and off. Each of us may be grateful for such buildings before we are through. As for those who have campaigned for the rights of gay and lesbian people, you may not feel personally involved in their cause, but somewhere among your children or grandchildren there may be someone who will be very grateful to them.

Anyone who has watched good advocates working with groups learns that they need to have known and trusted faces. They have to *be* there – becoming familiar figures in the hospital, the day centre or wherever the group gets together, and responding helpfully to anyone who wants to talk, not just dropping in for a weekly meeting and disappearing again. This kind of support takes time to build and is expensive to sustain, but it is enormously valuable. It also calls for a constant awareness of the boundary line between friendship and advocacy. Towards the end of a recent meeting a woman with Down's syndrome turned suddenly and spontaneously to the advocate helping the group, put an arm round her, and said, "You're our mum". "If that means you trust me to help you", the advocate replied "that's fine. But do remember, this is your meeting, not mine."

In the longer run, the causes that groups of this sort campaign for depend for their success on widespread public sympathy. It took 13 years for the Edinburgh Users Forum and some progressive professionals to secure the Crisis Centre they felt their city needed. It took only a few months for the new Scottish Parliament to make big reductions in fees for university students and charges for older people in need of care – both vastly more expensive projects. People coping with mental crises are not a small group. Most of us, at some stage of our lives, will know someone close to us who is going through this kind of experience. But they do not attract the public sympathy that people feel for students and older people.

Can advocacy of the kinds we have described help to build a new society that might be described as having 'a new "we"', in which people with mental and learning difficulties play their full part? Whereas they used to be hidden away by their families, such people are now increasingly 'coming out' to claim their rightful place in the world. This, not just the few, hard-fought victories it can win, is what group advocacy is really about.

That is what makes one of CAPS' latest projects so important. It has secured funds that will enable it to create an archive on paper, disk and film that records and celebrates the achievements of mental health service users in Edinburgh and the surrounding area– an archive, to be called "Oor mad history", which should interest and inspire people in many countries.

We have to think again about the meaning of 'community care', which is too often interpreted as professional services delivered to people living in their own homes – not as care in which the whole community is involved. That poses challenges we return to in the final chapter of this book.

SIX

Setting up an advocacy project and running it

Scott Rorison

Independent advocacy takes off

In Scotland, as elsewhere, advocacy projects usually emerged from organisations that gave a voice to people for whom they were already providing other services. ENABLE Scotland (formerly the Scottish Society for the Mentally Handicapped), Alzheimer Scotland – Action on Dementia, the Scottish Association for Mental Health and several smaller regional associations each gave birth to advocacy initiatives, working mainly with users of their broader range of services.

This pattern has been repeated in other parts of the United Kingdom and beyond. In the Republic of Ireland, for example, where advocacy is still in its infancy, the lead is being taken by long-established social care organisations such as the Brothers of Charity and Cheshire (Ireland).

Even where new advocacy agencies were set up, as they were under the Scottish Mental Health Act of 2003, with the sole purpose of providing advocacy services, it was likely that they would need a bit of time to find their feet and become fully independent. In some cases such agencies were 'hosted' by existing voluntary organisations, which helped them to set up a management structure, accounting and payroll services, banking facilities and insurance cover, and to gain charitable status. The agency that has provided much of the material for this book followed this path. It was at first managed by a national voluntary agency until it could find its own feet as a not-for-profit company with its own manager and board of directors. Other Scottish agencies will have developed in different ways, but all will have been shaped by broadly similar political and legislative influences peculiar to Scotland over the last decade.

Since the late 1990s, the UK government and, following the devolution of powers, the Scottish Executive have sent out guidance to local councils and the NHS on the commissioning and development of advocacy services. In 2000 this guidance was further strengthened when the Scottish Health Minister, Malcolm Chisholm, required local councils and health boards to jointly produce a 'three year plan' for the development of independent advocacy services in their areas. This raised the profile of advocacy and pushed it up the agenda of the public services that would have to commission and pay for it. It also led, in most areas, to an increase in the levels of investment being made in this service. Prior to this there were still some local authority areas in Scotland where no advocacy was available.

These developments hastened the emergence of a more unified advocacy movement in Scotland with the launch of Advocacy 2000, later replaced by the Scottish Independent Advocacy Alliance – both of them national umbrella groups speaking for local advocacy agencies. The Alliance and its forerunner, Advocacy 2000, undertook important work, with funding from the Scottish Executive, to map advocacy provision across Scotland and to develop a set of 'principles and quality standards' for advocacy organisations. While these principles and standards were being debated, discussions about the independence of advocacy took centre stage. Many of the people who would be clients for advocacy also relied on other services, such as residential care and day support services, which were offered by the same organisations that hoped to provide advocacy.

A clear distinction began to emerge between *independent* advocacy and other kinds of advocacy, with government guidance and local planning and investment being increasingly targeted to the independent version. Agencies and individuals involved in advocacy, while mindful of the importance of psychological independence, had been less concerned about structural independence. But from this point it became essential for advocacy agencies to be structurally independent, which meant doing nothing but advocacy, if they were to secure support from the state.

This emphasis on structural independence had a big impact on those involved in the management of these agencies. People who had previously been responsible for managing advocacy within an agency doing many other things found themselves responsible for running an independent voluntary agency.

Much of their work would be familiar to managers of any organisation. This chapter focuses on some of the issues that will particularly concern those who set up and manage an independent advocacy agency.

Getting started

The first task they all had to deal with – and must always continue to deal with – was to set up a constructive relationship with those who commission and fund their work. Understandably, those responsible for commissioning services on behalf of the public want to know, fairly precisely, what they will be getting for their money. How many bed spaces will be provided? How many hours of care and support will be made available? How many training placements will be completed?

Advocacy agencies present some challenges for evaluators. They cannot and should not be assembled in some kind of identikit fashion. Each will differ, depending on a whole range of factors, such as the kinds of places in which it operates, the resources at its disposal, the people it seeks to support and the models of advocacy it aims to practise. Rather than trying to impose some preconceived model of what an advocacy agency should look like, it will be more helpful if those commissioning advocacy services allow those responsible for developing them to adopt a community development approach. This means they will be guided by the views and priorities of local people, including those who may rely on their services. They will try to harness the knowledge and skills of local service users and others throughout the community. In this way, new projects can develop more organically, genuinely reflecting the needs and priorities of the people they represent and the communities they serve. Thus agencies will gain stronger roots in these communities. This approach will take longer, but is more likely to succeed in the long term. It requires those who commission the work to adopt new approaches, to take some risks and to show a high level of trust in the people they are dealing with. There will inevitably be different views among those involved about the purposes of the whole enterprise. Those differences need to be recognised, discussed and some workable agreement arrived at.

Most people think they know what advocacy is, but it means different things to different people. This is as true of professionals working in the health and social care services as it is for everyone else. Problems can arise when commissioners have expectations about the role of advocates that are at odds with the principles of this movement. It is asking a lot of statutory services to fund agencies that may use their money to support individuals and groups who are in conflict with those same services. This can prove particularly problematic when the things these individuals or groups ask for seem to the funders unrealistic or even totally unreasonable. Advocacy agencies have to stress that it is not their job to tell people what to do or to pass judgement on the views of the people they represent. It will require a strong commitment to advocacy and a good understanding of it on the part of funders if they are to support these agencies without fouling up their relationships with them.

Most people in Scotland would accept that understanding and awareness of the role of independent advocates has improved, at least among stakeholders working in services such as health and social work with whom they are most likely to come into contact. This has taken time and effort on both sides. The most effective advocacy agencies have had to work hard to establish a reputation for adopting a reasonable and constructive approach, seeking resolution rather than conflict whenever possible, but at the same time maintaining their independence and a commitment to their principles in all the work they undertake. Only through the development of a shared understanding of the role of independent advocacy can effective relationships between advocacy agencies and their commissioning bodies be maintained.

One of the advocacy agencies contributing to our research found that relationships with the commissioners of a new and innovative project providing independent advocacy for parents and carers of children and young people needing additional support for learning have been more difficult than those with longer established commissioners such as the health and social work services. That, they believe, may be due in part to a poorer understanding of the role of advocacy among professionals working in education and children's services than the understanding achieved among their colleagues in health and adult social work services. The same agency reports that joint training initiatives – on recent legislative developments for example – in which education, health and social workers have participated together have helped to break down barriers and promote a more constructive working relationship.

Maintaining independence

In the first version of 'principles and standards' for independent advocacy that was drawn up in Scotland, with leadership from Advocacy 2000, considerable emphasis was placed on the need for advocacy agencies to avoid conflicts of interest. It was suggested that one of the indicators that would show whether this was being achieved was the absence of any close relationships between those employed by advocacy agencies and individuals employed by local authorities, the NHS, or organisations engaged in the provision of services on their behalf. If that rule had been rigorously followed, in a country where so many people are employed by the NHS, local authorities and organisations delivering services on their behalf, advocates would have had to be pretty isolated and lonely people! More recent versions of the 'principles and standards' have concentrated more on the wise management of conflicts of interest than on unrealistic efforts to avoid them.

The character and purpose of advocacy makes it inevitable that those who do it will regularly be in conflict with those responsible for local authority and NHS services. That poses questions about the most appropriate channels for funding it. Some have suggested that the potential conflicts of interest that must arise when advocacy is funded through health and social work services could be averted if funds came directly from the government or through an agency or trust set up for the purpose.

While the present funding arrangements continue, advocacy agencies should try to secure support through a number of different funding sources. That may help to strengthen their psychological independence. But it will not be easy to arrange without becoming increasingly dependent on short-term grants that can be withdrawn at any time – not a good foundation for independence.

Recruiting people

The selection and recruitment of good people is the key to the success of any organisation. Independent advocacy agencies have to recruit not only employees but also volunteers, and people who will help to govern them by serving as board members and committee members. The best agencies will want to ensure that people who use or may want to use their services are meaningfully involved at every level of the organisation.

There is nothing new about advocacy. It is something that has always gone on in virtually every community, long before the emergence of formal agencies providing this service. Most communities contain individuals who probably do not describe themselves as 'advocates' but are well known for the help they give to people in trouble with authorities of any kind. Some advocacy agencies have found that, by seeking out these people and harnessing their skills, experience and connections, they have been able to tap into a valuable pool of expertise.

Our research on volunteers, reported in the next chapter, suggests that many of those who become involved as volunteers with advocacy agencies will already be actively engaged as community activists in other capacities. Experience suggests that lots of those who are attracted to advocacy work are motivated by their own experience of health and community care services, as workers in the field, or as users of services, or as carers, friends or relatives of those who have had to rely on these services. While this undoubtedly has its benefits it also brings with it some risks. Some people see advocacy as an opportunity to 'have a go at the system' or to 'settle old scores'. If they are to become wise and effective advocates they will need to be supervised sensitively, and carefully matched with clients to ensure they are not working on agendas of their own.

Training and accreditation

Professions normally require that their members hold recognised qualifications. This is thankfully not the case with independent advocacy, as we explain in Chapter Eight. In Scotland, few advocacy agencies view professional qualifications as essential requirements in a 'person specification' for most of their posts. While, as in all fields of work, training and practical experience have undoubted advantages, they can also have their downside. Long experience of a service system can encourage people to accept its routines and its hierarchies. Sometimes those with no experience of these systems, seeing things from a fresh perspective, will be more likely to challenge established practice. The volunteer advocate in a packed meeting of professionals will sometimes be the person who asks the obvious but neglected question, or challenges unquestioned assumptions that need to be re-examined.

Those who govern the work of advocacy agencies, as directors or members of a board or management committee, will collectively require a wide range of skills and experience. Not only will they be responsible for setting the strategic objectives of the agency and overseeing the quality of its work, they will also have to act as responsible employers, and ensure that substantial amounts of public money are put to appropriate and effective use. To bring together this complex mix of skills and interests can be a difficult task. It won't be achieved overnight. Some of those who know a lot about advocacy will have to learn to manage people and resources. Some of those who know a lot about management will have to learn more about advocacy.

The involvement of people who have direct experience of using health and community care services is likely to provide important insights that help other members of a board to keep focused on the core values that should underpin their work. If the danger of tokenism is to be avoided, however, it will be important to remember that some board members may require additional support to do their job. This will involve producing minutes and other documents in clear and simple forms; support that helps people to prepare for meetings; special transport arrangements for people with disabilities; constant encouragement to participate fully and in meaningful ways; and the pacing of meetings in ways that give people regular opportunities, every hour or so, for rest and recuperation.

It is important, we believe, to ensure there is a steady turnover of directors and executive committee members. Board members should serve for no more than five years. If they are allowed to continue for too long that discourages others from coming in to help, and reduces the pressure on directors and managers to find successors for them. No matter how able they may be, rule by a small oligarchy eventually stunts the depth and breadth of the agency's roots in the communities it serves. Directors who reach their retirement dates should be invited to stay in touch, to help as volunteers and eventually to rejoin the board.

Directors and their managers have to develop a quite sophisticated mutual appreciation of the scope and the limits of their roles. The board's most important task is to pick a good manager when the occasion for that comes; then to help him or her do a good job. That means they must be prepared to question the manager and senior staff about the work of the agency, the flow of funds required for it, policies governing the treatment of staff and any new commitments the agency may be contemplating. They should do their best to satisfy themselves that the work is being managed responsibly, effectively and humanely, with proper regard for the needs of its clients, its paid and volunteer workers and its commissioners. That is a formidable list of responsibilities. It must stop short of any attempt to manage the agency in a 'hands-on' way. That is the manager's job. A board that fails to question their manager and form their own views about important decisions, and a board that tries to micromanage their agency, intervening in detailed decisions about its daily work, are both failing in their duties.

As they grow in size and confidence, all voluntary organisations are in danger of losing touch with those engaged in the front-line work of their service. The agency from which much of our evidence comes has sought to counter this danger by including in its work people who use, or have used, its services – on panels interviewing candidates for jobs, for example. It also makes sure there are always volunteer advocates and a member elected by its staff on its board.

Support for advocates

When staff and volunteers have been recruited, it is important to ensure that they are well supported and supervised. This task of supervision is practised by managers in every kind of organisation. Supervisor management is concerned with establishing the accountability of workers to their organisation – ensuring that they do their jobs to a standard set by the organisation, that they attend on time, keep appointments and adhere to the policies of their employer; and ensuring, too, that good work is recognised and properly rewarded. In these respects, supervision in an advocacy agency is no different from that which should be found in any organisation that employs people.

There is also a second kind of supervision, more needed for those engaged in advocacy or similar tasks. It is based on a recognition that this kind of work can be particularly stressful, relying as it does on the personal qualities that an advocate brings to bear and the relationships they have with clients who may be vulnerable, challenging or, at times, seriously unwell. Advocacy is not a mechanical task, but one that relies on the constant use of personal skills in situations that often involve highly charged emotions. Therefore those involved in advocacy should be able to get regular and effective support. Many of the situations they encounter will be complex – sometimes unique. There will often be no 'right' answers to their dilemmas. They need an opportunity to reflect on their work, learn from their successes and failures, and cope with the emotional stresses involved.

This support can come from a variety of sources. Formal support from line managers can play an important part, but it can also be helpful if advocates have regular opportunities to talk with an outsider experienced in this kind of work. A volunteer recently retired from a career in an appropriate profession may be well placed to provide this kind of help. It can also be helpful to meet with colleagues doing similar work in their own and other agencies. In some areas local 'advocacy support groups', meeting regularly to discuss the dilemmas arising from their work, have proved an effective means of providing mutual support. Advocates meeting to present and discuss the cases in this book found the experience helped them in their work, and have asked that these discussions be continued. The fact that these meetings, like those of advocacy support groups, are non-hierarchical – no one is being evaluated or ranked in any way – is an important part of their character.

Giving this kind of support to volunteers can be even more difficult. The amount of time committed by volunteers, their level of experience and the complexity of the casework in which they are involved will vary widely. So too, therefore, will be the supervision they need. There will sometimes be practical difficulties if, for example, volunteers are in full-time paid work and cannot meet regularly with those expecting to supervise and coordinate their work during regular office hours. Supervisors will have to adapt their own hours if these people are to get the supervision they are entitled to. It will be important to ensure that volunteers are allocated sufficient work to keep them occupied and challenged, but not so much that they become overwhelmed by it. They may find that they are more exposed than paid staff are to deliberate attempts by those with whom they come into conflict to denigrate their professionalism, their expertise and their status. They need help if they are to cope with these rejections – help to recognise that such attempts to humiliate them are also directed at the clients (the patients!) who sought their help. Such behaviour explains why Parliament decided that people depending on the public service professions need the support of advocates.

Unmet needs

Those who are attracted to work in advocacy tend to be genuinely concerned about social justice and the welfare of vulnerable people. They want to uphold the rights of those who are most excluded from society's mainstream. The nature of their work means that they will often come into contact with people who are overwhelmed by their circumstances and at the end of their tether. But all advocacy agencies have limited resources of manpower and time. Deciding whom to help and whom to put further down the queue can be painfully difficult. There is a real danger that committed advocates will try to do more than is reasonable with the time and resources available to them. Helping them to say 'no' is another function of sensitive supervision.

The demand for independent advocacy is potentially huge. The new Mental Health Act in Scotland established a right to independent advocacy for everyone with a 'mental disorder' and we know that one in four of the population are likely to experience mental health difficulties at some stage during their lives.

The most successful advocacy agencies will find that more people seek their help than they are able to support. This means that difficult decisions have to be made about priorities. There will be differing views about how the queue for help should be ranked. Commissioners of services will want to ensure that those subject to interventions under the Metal Health Act, or other legislation on which their performance is to be assessed, are given priority. Meanwhile, advocates may know of potential clients who are not subject to such interventions but are in greater need of treatment and advocacy than those who are getting these things.

Picking the criteria to be used in deciding priorities will always be difficult. They will include: the urgency of a problem, the severity of its consequences for the client, the level of someone's vulnerability and the extent of their isolation. Whether the probability of a successful outcome should play any part in these decisions poses interesting questions, not least because someone whose case is lost and defeated may nevertheless feel empowered by being supported to participate in discussions and decisions that affect them.

Some advocacy agencies have been worried by the fact that it is those people who are best supported, best informed and most aware of their rights who are more likely to seek the help of an independent advocate. Meanwhile, as the demand for advocacy grows, the agencies providing it find that they have less and less time to seek out those who are most isolated, most vulnerable and least informed about their rights – the very people who probably have greatest need of advocacy. We return to these problems in our final chapter.

SEVEN

Volunteers

Introduction

The agency whose advocates provided most of the examples discussed in the last three chapters is typical of Scotland's advocacy services in relying on volunteers to do a lot of its work. Four of the clients described in earlier chapters were represented by volunteers. Some volunteers join the paid staff for temporary spells to fill gaps in the service that arise when paid workers are on leave or off sick and some of them move into paid jobs when the agency can recruit more staff. Meanwhile, some paid staff work as volunteers for other agencies. So there is no clear-cut distinction between the two.

Much of the advocacy already going on in Scotland before this service was set up by the Mental Health Act of 2003 had always been done by volunteers. The new service could not have got going so quickly without their help. Moreover, in remote and sparsely populated places – on islands, for example, where there may be no more than one or two people a year asking for an advocate's help – it will always be difficult to offer a service provided by paid staff. It is much better to train and support local volunteers. We believe there are more reasons why volunteers should always play a large part in our work – reasons that will become clear later in this chapter. Thus the service cannot be properly described without explaining how these volunteers are recruited, trained and supported in their work. As we explore these things we will find that they pose larger questions about a society's capacity to respond to the needs of its most vulnerable citizens.

How we made a study

The agency providing the evidence for this Chapter had, by the year 2007, trained more than 400 people in short courses, each lasting for about half a day every week for five or six weeks. These courses, taught by the agency's more experienced advocates, had been offered over the previous eight years in seven different places scattered across its large territory. (To drive from one end of it to the other takes about three hours.) 'Students' were recruited to these courses on a first come first served basis, with no promise that they would become advocates and no obligation to accept if they were invited to do so. That would be a separate and later decision, depending on the agency's gradually expanding needs and the wishes of those who had learnt something about its work.

The agency's board was aware that a few of its volunteers had given the agency a lot of help, but most of those taken on had given up the work fairly soon. In order to improve the whole system, it decided it needed to learn more about the experience these people had gained from its training courses and later as advocates. We think it is worth presenting the findings of the study it made, not because general conclusions can be drawn from so small a survey, but because it poses interesting questions and illustrates the kind of self-evaluation that agencies of this kind should carry out from time to time.

Questions put to those who had taken volunteer training courses were prepared and discussed with two groups of former students – 'focus groups' they were called – in different and contrasting places. These groups were asked to improve the questions and add some more.

The questionnaire produced in this way was then sent to the 277 people who had taken the courses and for whom the agency still had addresses, with a letter asking them to send back their answers along with any other comments they would like to make. It was not surprising that the agency had lost touch with many of those who had taken courses spread over eight years. One follow-up letter was sent to those who did not reply, and 99 completed and usable questionnaires were eventually returned. That was a response rate of 36%, which is not bad for surveys of this kind.

One of the last questions asked was, "Would you like to come and discuss a first draft of our report?" And 52 people said they would like to do so. A lot of these people came, along with staff and directors of the agency, to discuss the draft at two meetings held in widely separated places.

We summarise the answers given to our questions in the pages that follow, adding quotations from the comments people made in their own words, which are often more interesting than box-ticking responses. At the end we offer broader conclusions that deal with the whole issue of volunteering in services such as this.

Our interpretation of the survey calls for some explanation. We received very encouraging comments on our courses from the groups who discussed the first draft of our questions, from later discussions of a first draft of this report and from most of those who responded to our questionnaire. But the people most likely to take part in a study of this kind will be those who were happiest to get involved with the agency. We believed that those who had a less happy experience would be less likely to respond. So we take special care to report the more critical things that some people said because we believe there must be others out there – missing from this survey – who feel the same way. But it should be remembered that most of the responses we received came from people who were happy with our courses and with their encounters with this agency.

In eight years – which is the time between the earliest and latest courses taken – a lot of things can change. People move away and we lose touch with them. Meanwhile, opportunities for paid work had improved across most of our territory. So we may have attracted rather different kinds of people as time went by. We therefore divided the questionnaires into two equal piles: those from the 49 people who took one of our courses before the year 2004 and those from the 50 who took their first course in 2004 or later. But when we compared them we found there were very few differences between their replies. We will note the few we discovered.

Table 7.1 shows where these people took their courses, represented here by numbers, and how many of them – more than half – later became volunteer advocates. All the places where we held courses are represented. In each place the dates of courses are widely scattered – no single year dominates any local group.

Table 7.1: Where their courses were held and how many became volunteer advocates

Location	Total	Of whom became volunteers
1	37	23
2	19	8
3	18	10
4	11	3
5	10	6
6	3	2
7	1	1
Total	**99**	**53**

Why do people take a training course for volunteer advocates?

This was our first question and Table 7.2 shows the numbers who ticked the replies we had prepared with the help of our focus groups.

Table 7.2: Why did you take a course for advocates?

I was curious	23
Always interested in this work	43
To help a friend or relative	5
To gain confidence	17
To give something back	39
Hoped it might help me find paid work	19

Those answering these questions were able to tick as many replies as they wanted. They averaged about one and a half replies each. Only one category showed differences between earlier and later students on the courses: among the more recent students, taking courses since 2003, 16 (or 32%) said they hoped it would help them find paid work, but only three (6%) of those taking earlier courses gave this reason.

However, we cannot be sure how important this difference in the period of recruitment really is. It may be that the more plentiful job opportunities available in recent years prompted more people to use the courses in this way. But a later question showed no significant differences between the numbers of earlier and later students who actually took on more paid or voluntary work since completing their courses. The difference may be partly due to the fact that, with more time passing, more of those who took the earlier courses in the hope of finding paid work had moved away (perhaps their jobs took them elsewhere) and they are therefore missing from our survey.

Other replies suggest that many of those who take our courses have long been interested in our work – they are 'natural advocates' perhaps. Many hoped the course would enable them to "give something back" to the community, to gain confidence and get more involved. The courses do more than prepare people for advocacy. They contribute to economic and social development across our territory.

It is clear too that a number of those who take our courses and some of those who become volunteers have themselves been users of the mental health services. We do not know how many – we did not ask – but we value their contribution. It should be a reminder that volunteers – all volunteers – must have readily available support if they find the work stressful.

The most common replies given by those who wrote in their own answers came from people who hoped the course would help them in the jobs they were already doing, or simply 'upskill' them a bit. Others wanted to help vulnerable people and 'the underdogs'. Many brought valuable experience to their courses from work in other fields, paid and unpaid. These are active citizens: more than half of them were currently engaged in other voluntary work. Others were involved in less formal kinds of community action. One said the main aim of his voluntary work was "to destroy capitalism".

What did people think of our courses?

We asked people to assess our courses in five different ways: was the course interesting; helpful; were their teachers expert; good teachers; and did the course cover "the kinds of things you wanted to learn"? In each case they were asked to ring one number, ranging from 1 (meaning "not in the least") to 5 (meaning "yes, very").

People tended to give similar numbers, high or low, in all their answers. So, rather than search for small differences between these questions which are unlikely to be significant, we added up the numbers given by each person to all five questions and divided them into three roughly equal groups: the 'A's giving the highest scores, totalling 24 or 25 (out of a maximum of 25); the 'C's giving the lowest scores (totalling 19 or less); and a middle group of 'B's lying between them (scoring between 20 and 23).

For the reasons we have explained we will give special attention to the low scorers, but we should remember that most of these were in the high teens – around 70% of the maximum possible – which isn't a disastrous result. Only seven out of 99 people gave us a score of less than 50%. 'A's and 'C's were scattered through different years and places. So no single course was a total disaster or a total triumph (see Table 7.3).

The comments people wrote in for themselves were often warmly positive. Others noted particular things they would have liked to learn more about: "more information about services", "more on body language", "… on mental health" and "more role playing". Then – looking ahead to working for the agency – there were those who said more should have been done to get people quickly into advocacy after completing the course and there should have been clearer warnings about the delays that would be involved. (Much of the delay was due

Table 7.3: Participants' satisfaction with their courses

	A	B	C
Course locations	Maximum		Minimum
	24-25	20-23	19 or less
1	17	16	4
2	6	7	6
3	5	2	11
4	4	5	2
5	0	1	9
6	3	0	0
7	0	1	0
Total	**35**	**32**	**32**

to the Disclosure Scotland checks, which are required before volunteers can be employed, but these are now completed more quickly.)

To respond to some of these demands we would have to extend the courses. These normally run for five or six sessions, each lasting for about three hours. We asked our former students if they would prefer something different and Table 7.4 shows that the great majority were happy with the present arrangement. This poses a dilemma: do we cover more of the things some of them would like to learn about? Or do we stick with courses of the length that suits most people best? It's a normal dilemma to face – good courses make their students want to learn more.

Table 7.4: Preferred length of the course

Was your course: About the right length	71
Too short?	11
Too long?	6
Other answers or none	11

The low scores at site number 5 (see Table 7.3 earlier in the chapter) pose questions the agency has now discussed with people from that area. Various factors were probably at work. The agency was compelled by scarcity of funds to close an office it had opened there in earlier, over-optimistic years. That provoked understandable local resentment. There may also be a more widespread sense of injustice and hostility towards people in more fortunate areas among folk who have to live in a place where they have to contend with greater isolation and a bleaker economic climate than any other part of our territory experiences.

The agency cannot change those things, but it should recognise and discuss these problems more frankly with local people.

What did they do next?

Most of those who responded to our survey – 84 of them – wanted to become volunteer advocates when they finished the course. Table 7.5 shows the reasons they gave.

Table 7.5: What most attracted you to advocacy?

Found the work interesting	40
It's an opportunity to "give something back"	30
It's what I've always done	11
Other answers or none	3
Total	**84**

The 15 people who did not want to become advocates were asked for their reasons too (see Table 7.6).

Table 7.6: Reasons why 15 people chose not to volunteer

Too busy at home	2
Too busy with other work	5
Felt advocacy was not for me	2
Didn't feel equipped for the work	3
Other answers or none	3
Total	**15**

Then there were those who did want to become volunteer advocates but did not in fact do so. Their reasons were much like those of the people who chose not to volunteer, except that some felt the agency had discouraged them (see Table 7.7).

Table 7.7: Reasons why 31 people who did want to become volunteer advocates did not do so

Family responsibilities	6
Other work demands	17
Had to move house	1
Agency gave no encouragement	7

We cannot tell whether the agency gave those in the last of these groups a deliberate brush-off or had no need for more volunteers at that time, or whether an opportunity to recruit good people was missed. It is tempting to suggest that the courses should teach that advocacy has to 'begin at home' – helping people to advocate more vigorously for themselves, not to wait on others to 'give them encouragement'.

It is the experience of the 53 people who did become volunteer advocates that poses some of the most important questions the agency has to reflect on. Four of them had done a great deal of work for the agency. Some of them had worked temporarily as paid, 'sessional' staff to help out at times when regular staff were off sick or overwhelmed by pressure of work. But most of our volunteers have acted in very few cases and many of them have now left the agency. Table 7.8 shows their answers to the question "Roughly how many cases have you dealt with?" Nearly two thirds of our volunteers have dealt with less than five cases. Some of these will in time do more, but many have left us.

Table 7.8: How many cases have our volunteers dealt with?

Under 5	5–9	10–13	15–19	20 or more	No answer	Total
34	10	1	0	4	4	53

We have always been convinced that it is worth training more people than we can recruit as volunteers – and, indeed, more than may feel able to join us. The decision to start work as a volunteer is a different matter, to be dealt with after the course is over. We believe these courses should make a contribution to public education about the needs and rights of the people we are trying to help. Some of our students were already working in social work and other public services. They made important contributions to the discussion and will now be better equipped to help their clients seek the support of advocates when they need it. But, if people helped by volunteer advocates are usually relying on someone who has dealt with less than five cases, this poses worrying questions. Most of us would be reluctant to entrust our lives to a surgeon who had performed the operation we needed less than five times.

Why did we lose so many volunteers?

We asked those who responded to our questions, "Did you get the support and advice you needed from our staff?" Their responses – using the same 1-5 scores – were broadly encouraging (see Table 7.9).

Table 7.9: Did you feel you got the support and advice you needed from our staff?

Not in the least	1	2	3	4	5	Yes, very much	No answer	Total
		1	7	8	13	20		4	53

Next we asked, "What more could we have done?" –offering them replies that discussion with our focus groups suggested they might want to use. They could tick as many of these as they chose (see Table 7.10).

Table 7.10: What more could we have done to give you greater help? (53 responses)

More training	11
More information	9
A mentor or personal supporter	8
More opportunities to meet other volunteers	17
Better support and supervision	13

Some of those saying that more support or a mentor would be useful added that the staff member coordinating their work had done an excellent job of this kind. There were other positive comments: "I really enjoyed doing the advocacy ... meeting the clients and being a bit helpful to them"; "I learnt to look at people differently ... to see different points of view".

Others made more critical comments. "The line became unclear as to whether one was an advocate or a befriender, which are two totally different things." "There appeared to be no awareness ... of the different approaches required when working with people who have learning difficulties and those with mental health problems." Volunteers coping with such dilemmas need skilled and sympathetic support.

In other cases more efficient coordination and advice seemed to be needed. For one volunteer, the work "became very stressful – the prime reason why I left the service. There was a time when I had four clients at the same time ... in three different places [her coordinator, we should add, said this could not be true] ... and when advice was needed it was not the sort I could use or understand." Meanwhile another person said "too many cases were handled by one person and this led to a lot of volunteers feeling passed by and then lost interest".

Some of these experiences were reflected in answers to the next question put to volunteers who had given up working for the agency: "What were your main reasons for giving up?" (see Table 7.11).

Table 7.11: What were your main reasons for giving up?

Insufficient cases to work on	7
Lack of support and advice	8
Started a job or new job	9
Family responsibilities	8

Other answers written in for this question mentioned practical problems such as illness and financial stresses that compelled people to give priority to paid work.

Our support for volunteers seems to have improved. Six of the seven who felt they were given insufficient cases to work on and six of the eight who felt they were given insufficient support and advice had taken their training before 2004. Later recruits – who were equally numerous – seem to have had a better experience.

To conclude on a more hopeful note, it was encouraging to find that 32 people not now working as volunteer advocates would consider doing so in future. If the agency could assure them opportunities for work that is skilfully supported and efficiently coordinated they could be a great asset to the service.

What else did they gain from their experience?

Finally, we asked a few questions about things these people gained from their involvement in advocacy and about other developments in their work – paid and unpaid – which had taken place since they took our courses. Using the responses suggested by our focus groups, and encouraging people to tick as many as they wished, we gained the results shown in Table 7.12.

Table 7.12: Ways in which experience of our courses and of advocacy work has been helpful

Better understanding of needs of people with mental disorders	41
Ability to help a friend or relative	17
Getting enjoyable paid work	9
Getting into other enjoyable voluntary work	6

Many people said they had taken on new or more demanding work – paid and voluntary. Others wrote of important lessons they had learnt about the needs of vulnerable people, and about the good and bad ways in which public services work.

One said, "I have recently started a university course reading mental health, which I would never have considered before getting involved in advocacy". Some had gone into full-time work in other advocacy agencies. One, working in the public services, said she had learnt "how important it is to listen". Another said, "I now refer people who need your help to you". One said she had become an "internal advocate" within her service for vulnerable people. Others had learnt harsher lessons: "I was appalled by ... the bureaucratic systems in place to make it ... difficult for people ... to have their voices and rights met".

Scotland, Britain and the rest of the world

The information in this chapter has been derived from one small study carried out by one small agency. We cannot draw conclusions from it to guide people throughout the world. It has been presented partly as an example of the kind of simple, self-critical research that an agency of this kind should carry out on its own operations from time to time. Nevertheless, it poses questions and suggests ideas that others may find interesting. Before turning our attention to that wider audience we pause to consider whether Scotland has special features that we should bear in mind.

An extensive comparison of work and pay in Scotland, London and the rest of England concluded that, at the end of the 1990s, the Scots "stay in jobs longer, are more likely to be covered by collective bargaining and are more likely to be employed in the public sector. A higher proportion holds a degree, but also a higher proportion has no qualifications at all."[1] These patterns reinforce each other: the public sector is more unionised, employs more graduates and offers more secure jobs than other employers. Some people have argued that by bulking so large in Scotland the public sector has also helped to restrict enterprise, and gives Scotland a slower growth rate and higher rates of unemployment and poverty. But to explore that controversial territory would call for another kind of book.

The distribution of incomes, both among the Scottish population and in the rest of Britain, grew dramatically more unequal during the last quarter of the twentieth century. But the Scottish population were somewhat less unequal than the rest of Britain by the end of that century. Growing inequality between households in Scotland owed a lot to increases both in the numbers of households in which no one is working (the 'job-poor') and the numbers in which all adults are working (the 'job-rich').[2] The unemployed in Scotland, concentrated particularly on Clydeside and other areas where manufacturing and mining industries have experienced disastrous decline, seem to be more excluded from the mainstream of society than they are in England.

However, the proportions of Scottish people and English people who are active in voluntary organisations are very similar. In both countries employed people and people with middling or higher incomes are most likely to take part in voluntary work. Unemployed people – particularly in Scotland – are least likely to do so, and retired people come somewhere between these groups.[3] Scottish volunteers are most likely to be found working for their churches, for children and young people, for people with disabilities and for health projects of various kinds.

Another study, comparing participation in voluntary associations across 36 democracies, shows that voluntary activities tend to increase as countries grow richer. How long they have had democratic governments is also important: Canada, Denmark, New Zealand and France have the highest participation rates; Bulgaria, Russia, Hungary and Poland the lowest. Britain lies close to the average, coming 15th out of 36 in the percentage of its people participating in voluntary associations.[4]

Summing up these comparisons, we can say that, although the Scottish economy has some distinctive features, Scotland's main patterns of voluntary activity seem to be much the same as those found south of the border. Meanwhile Britain's involvement in voluntary work seems broadly typical of the middle range of democracies. So the conclusions that follow, which go beyond the findings of our survey to draw on our general experience of working with volunteers, may interest others besides the agency for which they were originally designed.

Conclusions

Throughout the community there are people with a generous capacity for voluntary action. Some of them are natural advocates, prepared to support vulnerable neighbours and capable of challenging the authorities on whom they depend; and some of these have been users of the services that advocates have to deal with. These are the people whose help an advocacy agency most needs and they respond readily to invitations to take courses that will equip them better for this work.

Our own advocates teach the courses we offer. Besides giving an initial training to people who may become volunteer advocates, they are an investment in social and economic development, enabling many of those who take them to do creative and fulfilling things they would not otherwise have done. They also help to make public services more humane and responsive.

But volunteers in this field, as in so many others, tend to be people on the move: men and women who have had to give up their jobs and are looking for new things to do; students who have completed academic courses and are preparing to enter the world of paid work; people who have had a spell of illness and are now seeking recovery, and the rebuilding of friendships and credibility; mothers who have for years been caring for children or older relatives, and are now liberated to return to wider worlds of voluntary and paid work – looking for contacts, recovering their confidence, and building a CV.

This means that many will use training courses of the kind we provide as a bridge to other things – not necessarily to advocacy. There will therefore be a pretty high turnover among those who join us. Only a minority will stay with us for a long time. We may, nevertheless, have offered them an experience they will make good use of.

Being so brief, our courses inevitably fail to cover many things that intelligent students would like to learn about. But they are also the right length for most of the people who take them. Few want a longer course. So tutors need to discuss the content of the course with their students as it unfolds and do their best to include things that most interest them – students and teachers shaping the course together (which is the way education should always work).

Advocacy is a new and demanding field, creating stresses and dilemmas of many kinds for those who work in it. They need skilled and sustained support, careful matching to clients and efficient coordination. It is unfair to them and their clients, and wasteful of the resources we invest in training them if we fail to give them that backup. Our agency seems to be getting better at this task, but needs to consider carefully how it can improve the support and management that volunteers and their clients should be entitled to expect.

It seems clear that the period between the point at which their courses end and the point at which volunteers have gained a good deal of practical experience is the crucial one for them – a time when some are lost before they get properly started and more are lost because they find the work too stressful or gain too little support and advice. This is the phase that an agency such as ours particularly needs to attend to, improving its arrangements in consultation with the volunteers themselves.

A training policy for volunteers should lead beyond the initial introductory course to give them opportunities for further training that will enlarge their understanding of the work and the people they work with. That policy should be part of a broader training strategy that also meets the needs of paid staff and board members.

Many volunteers say they would find it particularly helpful to have more frequent contact with other volunteers doing similar work. We have in fact tried to arrange that, but attendance at such gatherings has not been good. Clearly such a policy needs to be planned more carefully if it is to succeed. We should try again, and make sure that these encounters are enjoyable as well as informative.

Before setting up more courses we should approach the considerable number of our former students and volunteers who say they would consider joining or rejoining our service, consult them about the arrangements that would best help them to do so and draw on this important potential resource. Some of them say they will need refresher courses before they get started.

Those in the public services that commission and pay for advocacy work also need to understand these things. Well organised and skilfully supported volunteers may not be cheaper than full-time paid staff. The arguments for recruiting, training and employing them are not mainly economic. Volunteers contribute things the paid professionals, on their own, are less likely to offer – such things as widespread influence and deeply rooted knowledge from within the community and its public services; a capacity to work in remote and sparsely populated areas where it would be uneconomic to employ paid staff; and a willingness to challenge professional and bureaucratic authorities arising from the fact that volunteers are more likely to have used the services themselves and are less likely to become accustomed to their practices and complacent about them.

Paid professional advocates have an equally important job to do. Recruiting, training and supervising volunteers, some of whom should have been users of the services that advocates are dealing with, are important parts of that job.

Most advocacy agencies do less training than we have done. Some of them claim to take more trouble over selecting the people who take their courses. We believe it is very difficult to forecast who will make a good advocate. Training and later experience change people – that's what education is *for*. So it is wiser to welcome all those to whom you can offer a place. They will probably make a better job of selecting themselves. Recruiting volunteer advocates is a later and separate step, which must of course be taken with great care.

We have focused this chapter on volunteer advocates, but there are many other tasks in which volunteers can help. An agency of this kind needs board members, researchers, personal supporters for individuals and groups, and experts on computing, book keeping, the law, the media and much else. It should ask its students and volunteers about their interests and skills, and discuss various ways in which they could help. Advocacy is a community-based movement, not just a professional specialism.

Notes

[1] Robert Elliott, Vania Gerova and Euan Phimister, 'Distribution and structure of pay', in John F. Ermisch and Robert E. Wright, *Changing Scotland*, Bristol, The Policy Press, 2005, p 180.

[2] David Bell and Gregor Jack, 'Income inequality', Chapter 9 in John F. Ermisch and Robert E. Wright, *Changing Scotland*, Bristol, The Policy Press, 2005.

[3] Jeanette Findlay and Patricia Findlay, 'Volunteering and organisational participation', Chapter 18 in John F. Ermisch and Robert E. Wright, *Changing Scotland*, Bristol, The Policy Press, 2005.

[4] Paul F. Whiteley, 'What makes a good citizen? Citizenship across the democratic world', Chapter 9 in Alison Park et al (eds), *British social attitudes,* London, Sage, 2008.

EIGHT

Making advocacy accountable

Why should advocacy be evaluated?

Every public service should be evaluated from time to time to make sure it is doing its job properly. But those paid by their fellow citizens to act as advocates for people who may be very frail and engaged in conflicts with powerful authorities have a special duty to show that they are doing their best to serve their clients in an independent, well-informed and skilful way, without conflicting interests. That duty weighs particularly heavily on them in Scotland where the agencies they work for usually have a monopoly of reasonably secure public funding for this kind of work in the territory they cover. Although their contracts could be transferred to other advocacy agencies at some rather distant point in the future, they are not exposed to the daily discipline of competing for customers in a market place. These are privileges that most voluntary agencies can only dream of.

People working in this field in England and Wales and in the US have prepared 'charters' and long lists of tests that advocacy agencies should pass to show they maintain proper 'quality standards'. They can afford to be rigorous because advocacy is growing slowly – usually for particular groups of clients in particular areas. Meanwhile the spokesmen of government, offering tempting hopes of more secure funding at some point in the future, have pressed advocates to organise training courses leading to accreditation – accreditation that would give successful candidates membership of a professional institute that would assure the world of their competence; accreditation that could also be withdrawn if they failed to maintain the proper standards. This has long been the route taken by public service professions – doctors, midwives, social workers and many others – to gain recognition and a place on the public payroll. Some advocates hope eventually to follow their example. Others have resisted that idea, arguing that advocates should not try to become a profession of that kind. We will discuss these arguments at the end of this chapter.

Scotland's way – so far

When the new Scottish government set up an advocacy service for people with mental health disorders under the 2003 Act, it did this by requiring local social work and health authorities to commission voluntary agencies to provide the service and get it up and running by October 2005. It also commissioned another voluntary body – the Advocacy Safeguards Agency (ASA) – to evaluate the work of each of the agencies that grew up to provide this service. There are various opinions about the competence of the ASA, but we need not go into that because the agency folded quite soon and has not so far been replaced. Instead, the government worked with the advocacy agencies and their Scottish Independent Advocacy Alliance to ensure that guidelines and standards for the work were prepared and published. (Their main report is due soon.) It would then be the duty of the local authorities and health boards paying for the work to satisfy themselves that these standards are maintained. With varying rigour these 'commissioners' of advocacy work, as they are called, already keep an eye on the service, but they have had more urgent things to do than evaluate it in any systematic way. Getting an independent evaluation of a new service is always difficult because the only people who have learnt enough to do the job properly will usually be working for the service concerned.

Hard-nosed bureaucrats may think this relaxed regime is irresponsibly tolerant. But it has made a lot of sense for the early years of this service, allowing the people involved in it to work out what its principles and practices should be. But that creative freedom will not last for ever. Sooner or later there will be scandal and a panic – advocates who appear to have abused their power, some horrible crime committed by them or by one of their clients, while newspapers and politicians mount a hue and cry about the service. There will then be senior members of other professions, as the example quoted in the Introduction to this book makes clear, who will not be sorry to see the whole project scuppered.

To provide a good service for the people they are trying to help, and to prevent disasters of this kind, advocates should be developing convincing ways of evaluating their work and presenting their findings to the various groups who have an interest in it. Having led the world in setting up free and independent advocacy for people with mental health difficulties, Scotland should also lead the way in evaluating this service. If we fail to do that, the service and those who depend on it will suffer.

This chapter is intended to help in that task. It does not produce yet another list of principles and targets. There are plenty of those already. It poses the questions that evaluators will have to think about. We believe there is no list of requirements – no single 'exam paper' – that every agency must 'pass'. The people they serve, their aims and methods, are too varied for that. This variety is not a problem. It should be encouraged, for it provides a launch pad for new developments that may in time prove fruitful. Advocacy should remain a broadly based movement, not a standardised service cast in a single bureaucratic mould. Advocates in each agency should think out for themselves the kind of evaluation that best suits their needs. We hope this chapter will help them to do that. We prescribe no list of indicators or targets that every agency should measure up to. Instead, we pose the more important questions each agency should be able to answer.

Accountability for what? And to whom?

Those who formulate principles and standards for advocacy usually divide their task into about three stages, starting with *principles*, which are "core beliefs about independent advocacy … the ideas that guide everything that advocates … do". Then come *standards*, which show what has to happen if these principles are to be applied. Finally there are large numbers of *indicators*, which measure how well advocacy agencies live up to these standards. This is the formula prescribed by *Principles and standards for independent advocacy*, a report published in 2008 that was prepared by the Scottish Independent Advocacy Alliance (SIAA) after consultations with the advocacy movement.

Two years before the SIAA's principles appeared, Action for Advocacy, an umbrella group speaking for advocacy agencies in England and Wales, published a similar statement: *Quality standards for advocacy schemes, based on The Advocacy Charter*. It formulated its arguments in much the same way, setting out a number of *principles*, and then, for each principle, presenting: (1) a *definition*, (2) a *rationale* explaining the reasons for it, (3) *standards* of practice, with examples, and (4) a *code of practice for advocates*.

It offers ten *principles*, which can be summarised in this way:

1   **Clarity of purpose**: "clearly stated aims".
2   **Independence**: ensuring "the advocacy scheme will be structurally independent from statutory organisations and preferably from all service provider agencies". (Scotland would have omitted the word "preferably".)

3 **Putting people first**: ensuring that advocates put the wishes of their clients first.

4 **Empowerment**: supporting "self-advocacy" and helping service users to "get involved in the running and management of the scheme".

5 **Equal opportunity**:"tackling all forms of inequality, discrimination and social exclusion".

6 **Accessibility**: the service must be "free of charge to eligible people" and do its best to make it easy for everyone to use it.

7 **Accountability**: ensuring there are good "systems for ... monitoring and evaluation of [the] work".

8 **Supporting advocates**: ensuring that they "are prepared, trained and supported" and have "opportunities to develop their skills and experience".

9 **Confidentiality**: calling for "a written policy on confidentiality ... and any circumstances under which confidentiality might be breached".

10 **Complaints**: ensuring clients have well-understood rights and procedures for making complaints about the service they get.

It is interesting that this document talks about 'schemes' for advocacy, not 'agencies' – probably for the good reason that the work goes on in all sorts of ways, not necessarily in an organisation set up for the purpose. We use the word 'agency' throughout this book because we are talking about advocacy that *is* conducted through an organisation that does this and nothing else – an organisation that ought to be accountable for what it does.

The principles set forth in these documents are excellent, leading to many practical proposals for putting them into practice and recording the standards to be achieved. Action for Advocacy rightly stresses that evaluations should be conducted by an agency that is independent of those whose work is to be evaluated. It warns agencies that this will be quite expensive and may produce disappointing results. So it has set out a three-stage process that would enable agencies to approach the examination cautiously and with better chances of success. Is there anything more to be said?

None of these documents, or their even more elaborate predecessors prepared by Americans, explains precisely to *whom* advocates should be accountable. Quite rightly, they focus mainly on accountability to the people whom advocates try to help. Without detracting in any way from that priority we should remember that others are involved in this service to whom advocacy agencies must also be accountable. Otherwise we may forget important things.

Other interests that must be considered are those of:

- **The authorities commissioning – paying for – advocacy work**. They are likely to want to know a few things about the board or management committee running the agency. They will also want to know how much they spend on direct services to individual clients, and how much is spent on other things such as campaigning work, overheads and the expenses of staff and board members. Money is scarcely ever mentioned in the prescriptions for evaluation we have so far been offered.
- **Staff and volunteers working for the agency**. Staff will want to know how their salaries compare with those of people doing similar work; whether they can rely on a decent pension at the end of the day; and what rights of appeal they will have if their work is condemned as a result of some evaluation. They and volunteer advocates will want to know what support they will receive in their work and what opportunities there will be for further training. They will also want to know what arrangements have been made to protect advocates working with clients who have a history of violence.
- **Managers and board members responsible for the general progress of the agency** will want to know how secure its income is; how many months they would have to close it down or find other sources of money if their present funders cut off all further support. The independence of an advocacy service depends heavily on the answers to these questions.
- **The community at large**. What the agency can do for its clients depends in the long run on the support and understanding these people receive from neighbours, fellow workers, local news media and the public at large. So questions must be asked about the steps taken by the agency to educate the public about the needs and rights of the people advocates are trying to help.

These thoughts threaten to produce a formidably long list of indicators. A list so long that no one responsible for a small agency, spending all its modest income on urgently needed advocacy, could deal with on a regular basis – particularly if it had to pay another agency to do the job. It is more important that evaluations be conducted frequently than that they cover everything it might be interesting to know.

It is also vital that the people most involved – particularly the staff – play a central part in working out how to evaluate their work. Each agency's aims – and thus its ways of monitoring its progress – will be a bit different, and should evolve and change in the course of time. If their staff feel they are being compelled to jump through hoops set up by distant bureaucrats, they will not take 'ownership' of any evaluation they have to undergo. They will be tempted to fake or fudge the results, or – worse still – to distort their work, not to serve their clients but to tick the right boxes and hit the targets. Doctors, social workers, teachers and other public service professions have in recent years had too much experience of these patterns.

So the suggestions that follow are deliberately stripped down to a realistic minimum. If hard-pressed advocacy managers groan in despair at the prospect of having to assemble this information, we will have failed because they will rightly conclude that it is more important to keep their service going and prevent waiting lists for it emerging. What we offer *are* only 'suggestions'. If practising advocates do not reshape them in various ways to suit their own agencies' needs, we will again have failed, for they will not have thought through this task or taken full ownership of the system it creates.

Evaluating advocacy

We have said that, besides the clients themselves, there are four broadly defined groups entitled to an evaluation of the service: the commissioners or paymasters; advocates and other staff; managers and their board or management committee; and the community at large. For practical purposes that is too elaborate a list and the things that each group needs to know will overlap a great deal. So, to simplify the task while trying to ensure that essentials are not forgotten, we focus on three standpoints from which advocacy should be made accountable. The approach we propose could apply equally well to almost any public service – a school, a hospital, a social work service – which suggests we have got the fundamental requirements for evaluation about right.

I Bottom-up accountability: to clients, their families and the public at large

These are some of the main questions an advocacy agency should be expected to answer for people viewing its work from these points of view:

(a) If someone needs an advocate, how do they find out about the service? How can they get its help?

(b) Having been referred to the service or made their own approach to it, how long do clients have to wait before meeting an advocate? Are there waiting lists for certain kinds of client? And which kinds? (For important parts of the work, such as representation at tribunals, delay would amount to refusal of service.)

(c) What rules does the agency follow to make sure that its advocates focus on responding to the wishes of their clients and are independent of other agencies they may have to deal with? As happens so often in these lists, the basic rules are fairly simple. The agency is securely funded for the work it has been asked to do and it does no other work. Advocates are well trained and have no compromising connections with people from whom their clients seek a response.

More interesting are the rules that apply when independence may be unavoidably compromised. In small communities, the families most likely to provide advocates are likely to be active in many other fields. Perhaps the advocate's husband or daughter works for the hospital or social work service from which the client wants action of some kind. Moreover, when work on the case begins it may be impossible to foresee that it will call for negotiation with a bank, a housing association or some other body the advocate has a connection with. What then? Is a potential conflict of interest carefully explained to clients – or their families or 'named persons' where necessary? Are they given the option of seeking the help of another advocate wherever that can be arranged?

What are the limits to the commitment of advocates to their clients? Do they explain to clients, when necessary, the reasons why they cannot break the law; and must not put them or other people in danger; or tell lies on their behalf?

(d) What rules assure clients that any information the agency gains about them will be treated as confidential and will be shared with others only if the client permits that? Again, the basics are obvious. But what are their limits? If the safety of someone – their own child perhaps – is endangered by clients' behaviour, will the need to seek help from protective services be frankly explained to them?

(e) Does the agency conduct feedback surveys of its clients from time to time to ask them what they think of the service they have received? Are these surveys conducted in ways that assure anonymity for those who respond to them? What use is made of the results? Are summaries of the findings presented in annual reports or in other ways?

(f) Does the agency work with groups as well as with single clients? That may not be possible for some types of client, in some kinds of places, or with some kinds of staff. But it is when users of public services come together to share the experiences they have had and begin working out how things could be improved that advocacy helps to change the world, rather than just helping individuals cope a bit more successfully with the world as it is. Advocacy offered only to individuals can too easily reinforce the idea that when things go wrong that will usually be the fault of a frail person who needs help to sort things out. Groups are more likely to remind us that when things go wrong that is too often because public services and other powerful bodies work in disempowering ways.

If the agency is working with groups, what precisely have they achieved? What steps are taken to ensure that they offer empowering experiences for their members, not just the cheerful activities that any day centre should provide for its users?

(g) What steps are taken to educate the community and its leaders about the needs of those whom the agency tries to help? Are community policemen, local councillors, members of our various parliaments and assemblies, and local journalists brought to meetings of various kinds with the agency's clients? Do they listen and respond in practical ways to what they hear and see?

Are groups of clients enabled to get out into the community to assert their needs and participate in its life – particularly its political life? Do staff and board members – as teachers, preachers, writers, community activists, etc – get out into the community to talk with local groups and speak at meetings of various kinds, telling them about the needs and rights of those whom their agency serves?

(h) There will always be people with urgent need of an advocate's help who never hear of the service and perhaps get no help from other public services they should be entitled to – homeless people, asylum seekers and returning service personnel for example. What steps does the agency take to get in touch with these people and help them? Does it help other agencies that may be in contact with them to provide advocacy services of their own?

Thoughtful advocates will want to add to these questions in ways that meet the needs of their particular clients and the area they serve – perhaps comparing the social character of those they help with that of the population at large. Are some groups being left out? They will want to record the problems coming up in their work so that they can take some of these up with managers of the services concerned. But rather than add to this list of questions, we should note some we have *not* asked.

We have not asked what proportion of their cases are 'won' by advocates. Agencies will naturally want to keep an eye on those achievements and congratulate the advocates responsible for them. But it would be a mistake to make a regular report with figures of this kind. Why? Because the capacity of psychiatrists to win their cases before tribunals may be due partly to the fact that they have learnt that good advocates will point out any weaknesses in their recommendations. Because we do not want to put advocates under pressure to turn down cases that are unlikely to be won. And because it is difficult to measure 'success'. Perhaps a client was, for the first time in their life, listened to and treated with respect. Was this as important as the outcome of the case? Was a skilled and committed advocate in fact convinced that a 'victory' for the client was likely to prove disastrous for them? (Disastrous, but it was what they wanted.) Would that be a 'success' – or just a job properly completed?

2 Top-down accountability: to officials of the commissioning agencies, the government, and ultimately to all of us as voters and taxpayers

These people will want to know the answers to many of the questions we have already asked. But they will also want to ask questions such as these.

(a) Is the agency's constitution available for inspection? What does it say about governance? For example, about access to membership of the society concerned, the size of its governing body, how that body is appointed and any restrictions on those entitled to belong to it? (Staff of the paymaster agencies should attend only as observers.) How are the agency's executive committee members selected and its officeholders chosen? How often does each of these bodies meet? Are there any restrictions on the periods for which people may hold office? (A regular turnover should be ensured.)

(b) More informally – because these things are unlikely to appear in the constitution – they should ask: what parts are played in the agency's membership and its governing body by users or former users of services for people with mental disorders? Do they serve, for example, on panels that interview candidates for jobs with the agency? (Generally good things to do.) Are members of the governing body or its executive committee related to the staff? (Generally not good.)

(c) How many individual and group clients does the agency currently have? Are these numbers going up or down? How do they divide into different groups – for example, people with mental health difficulties, people with learning disabilities, older and frail people, and people with other kinds of needs that will vary from one agency to another? Does this distribution fit with the agency's stated aims and with the general expectations of those who pay for it all? How much of the work is done by trained volunteers and how much by paid advocates?

(d) What is the agency's annual income and expenditure? Where does the money come from? How have these figures changed in recent years?

How is expenditure divided between the direct costs of the service provided, and overhead costs for administrative staff and premises – payments that have to continue, whatever the current output of services? (Heavy overhead expenditure would call for some explanations.)

What is the salary of the highest paid member of staff? And the lowest paid members? How much is spent on the expenses of staff and board members?

(e) Bringing evidence from questions (c) and (d) together, what is the average gross cost and the direct cost (not counting overheads) of each case – or each of the main types of case – that the agency deals with? Are these average costs going up or down? (As a new service expands and gains experience of the work, costs per case should be falling.) Are volunteer advocates cheaper than paid staff, when account is taken of the costs of training, recruitment, support, and their expenses for travel, postage and telephones?

(f) Are there significant differences in the money received and the money spent in different parts of the agency's territory? Can these be explained by differences in the resources, the generosity or the policies of different local authorities and health boards, or in other ways?

There will be other questions that many would add to this list – perhaps about the size, density and social composition of the population to be served (thinly spread populations are more expensive to reach; older populations more likely to suffer dementia), or about the numbers of mental hospitals there are in the area and the numbers of in-patients they hold (giving rise to more tribunal work). But these should be for each agency to decide for itself.

3 Accountability to the governors, manager and staff of the agency itself

These people will be interested in all the questions we have suggested, but will want to add a few more for their own purposes.

(a) How much money – measured as months of current expenditure – does the agency maintain as a minimum reserve?

(b) If all further funding, beyond that already promised, were to be cut off, how long would the governing body have to raise further money or to wind up the agency before closing it down?

(c) The most important asset that any enterprise has is its own staff. A modest but significant proportion of its expenditure should be devoted to the professional development of these people through training courses, attendance at conferences and 'away days', a small library, and so on. There should be a policy giving all staff well-understood rights to participate in these things and an obligation to share what they learn with colleagues when they return to base. If all the money goes on direct service to clients, a downward spiral of growing exhaustion and declining morale will set in.

(d) Staff should be entitled to contracts, rates of pay, expenses and pensions that compare fairly with those of people doing similar work in other public services. They should also have: the right to regular, helpful meetings with their line manager; well-understood procedures for dealing with disciplinary matters and complaints (about them or from them); the right to belong to a trade union; an elected observer to speak for them at board meetings; and protection from discrimination on any of the grounds dealt with by equal opportunities policies.

(e) Staff and volunteers working for the agency should be assured that it has a policy for the management of risk that will help to protect them and others if they are dealing with people who have a record of violent behaviour or of self-harm. They should play a part in formulating and occasionally reviewing this policy.

Again, there are more questions that will interest people viewing the agency from this standpoint, but we should leave them to develop this list in ways that suit their own needs. As before, some of our omissions have been deliberate. We have not asked how many staff are professionally qualified. It is helpful if some of them and some board members have good qualifications and experience of various kinds – as nurses, social workers, lawyers, accountants or managers, for example. But, for reasons we explain in the next section, we do not believe that all advocates should be formally qualified for their work.

Accreditation

We promised to come back to the question of accreditation at the end of this chapter. Other professions have devised their own training – starting in universities and colleges, and completed in prescribed periods of practice under supervision in various professional settings. Advocates deserve similar opportunities.

Do we need to go further? This kind of training usually gives successful candidates membership of a professional institute, association or 'college' which has a responsibility to monitor standards of practice and to discipline members who fail to maintain these standards – excluding them from practice altogether in the worst cases. There are many in the advocacy movement – particularly in England and Wales – who would like their profession to evolve in this customary way.

Scotland has rejected that policy. There, most people believe that proper accreditation is necessary, but it should apply to agencies, not to individuals. This is also the policy of the Scottish Independent Advocacy Alliance.

Once you set up a nationwide service, as Scotland has done, rather than a scatter of precariously funded 'schemes', you have to recognise that it will for many years be impossible to insist on formal qualifications for all advocates. Training courses do not develop until there is a predictable demand for them – and then only get going when there are enough teachers with good experience of the work, and sufficient research has been done and published to give them and their students a literature to read.

These things will develop during the coming years. Books like this one are intended to carry that process forward. Training courses and practice teachers will then need to evaluate their students' work and decide who passes appropriate examinations, which of them do so with distinction, what can be done for those who fail, and so on. That provides a necessary evaluation of their teaching. (How much did their students learn?) Students, too, are entitled to a record of their achievements – something to add to their CVs.

That is all right and proper. But governments and some professional leaders like to go further than this and compel all who claim to work as members of a profession to secure and maintain registration by an accrediting body. This brings many advantages. There are mechanisms – through journals, conferences and research groups – to advance and disseminate knowledge. Bad practitioners can be struck off and excluded from the work. And the profession's leaders, controlling access to their ranks, win a monopoly that helps to protect their members' terms of service and increase their incomes. (If there are unemployed doctors because medical schools are producing too many graduates, this is called a problem of 'oversupply' and entry to the schools is restricted. It is never a problem of overpayment of doctors or underfunding of health services.)

But the interests of those who depend on the profession's services and the community at large that pays for it all are too often neglected. That's why advocacy came into being in the first place. As the public service professions came to power, protected by some of the most powerful institutions in this country's 'establishment' – royal colleges, trade unions and universities, along with the forces of local government and the civil service – the people depending most heavily on their services, including many with no organisation to speak for them, were too often neglected or exploited.

The advocacy service, which has been set up as one part of society's response to this imbalance of power, needs and values the qualified and experienced professionals it has been able to recruit – former nurses, social workers, managers and others. But many of its advocates – staff and volunteers alike – came into this work without formal qualifications of any kind. They joined because they have always been natural advocates, prepared to help anyone suffering neglect or injustice; because they have themselves had to depend on public service professions whose humanity and competence could not always be relied on; or because they have for years cared for their frail parents or children, and had to learn how to fight for their rights.

If some officials and some members of long-established professions view these 'unqualified' advocates (and perhaps their accents and their general style) with suspicion or distaste, that explains why we need advocacy to support those who depend on the services of such people. If advocates qualified only by long and hard experience were to be excluded from the work, we would have to start all over again – setting up a new movement, prepared independently to speak to power on behalf of the powerless.

NINE

Roadblocks

The problem

Cases discussed in previous chapters show that advocates will sometimes come up against public services which, despite the advocates' best efforts, completely fail to give their clients the help they are entitled to expect. That may be because they have run out of money, because they are badly managed, because they are hostile to the client, because they have chosen to focus on other priorities or for other reasons. It is unfair to advocates, and useless for their clients, to send them out to ask for things we know will be refused. But advocates would be failing in their duty if they accepted bad services without trying to make them better. So what should they do?

There can be no single answer to that question – what can be done will depend on local circumstances. But this chapter may help people who encounter such roadblocks to formulate a policy for dealing with them. A policy of some sort will certainly be needed.

Advocates may, in their own time, be active in all sorts of causes. But the agencies they work with have to accept that they cannot be all-out campaigners – constantly writing letters to the press, seeking the help of politicians and staging demonstrations in the street. The authorities paying for their work would be entitled to say: "We pay you to advocate for your clients; not to light fires under us." More important still, they would find their campaigns sometimes divide the clients for whom they claim to speak. Some parents of children with additional educational needs passionately believe their youngsters should go to schools outside the mainstream. Others believe, equally passionately, they should go to mainstream schools. Some patients would resist electro-convulsive therapy at all costs. Others find it helpful. Advocacy agencies cannot campaign for both. So what else should they do?

Principles and practice

First, some guiding principles. We should start with the users of our services, find out what they want and help them to campaign for those things when they wish to do so. We speak for them and for no one else. If we do get involved in protests we should involve our clients, their friends and families in any way we can.

We should always begin in a low-key, polite fashion and remain courteous but firm, even when we have to jack up the pressure. We should try sympathetically to understand the problems that public services have to contend with and work towards solutions that do not humiliate anyone, while always remembering they are *their* problems, not ours. Our first concern must be with our clients' problems.

In more practical terms, this means we should:

1   Help and support service users who wish to bring about improvements in the services they depend on. Their voice is harder to disregard than ours because they have personal experience of the things they are talking about. And they all have votes.

    For example, with some help from one of our advocates, groups of people with learning disabilities have joined campaigns to prevent the closure of their local hospital. Smaller examples are important too. One of these groups invited their community policeman to their meetings, persuaded him to put a parking ticket on cars parked in dangerous places outside their day centre and asked him to get the white lines on the road repainted yellow, which will enable the police to charge the drivers who disregard them. White lines, he explained, are 'advisory', but yellow lines have the force of law.

2   Advocates themselves – or their line managers – can approach the directors and managers of failing services and ask them to do better, bringing users of their services with them whenever they can. It may be helpful to draw their attention to better practice that is to be seen in neighbouring authorities. Where the targets of their appeals are voluntary or commercial services they can seek help from the public authorities that pay for them.

3   In some cases, clients will have a good legal claim – over discrimination they have experienced or a care assessment to which they are entitled, for example. It may be useful to seek the help of a good solicitor.

4   Advocacy agencies can approach national bodies supervising the services they are concerned about and seek their help – the Mental Welfare Commission in Scotland, for example; or ombudsmen of various kinds.

5   They can approach, or set up, voluntary groups – a local mental health forum, for example – that bring together services speaking for people who face similar problems and ask them to take the

matter up. That may give them strength in numbers, ensuring that no single agency has to take all the flak. As a postscript to this chapter we briefly describe the work of GAIN – the Gateshead Advice and Information Network – which is an encouraging example of a local body of this kind.

6   There are national bodies like ENABLE Scotland for people with learning disabilities, the Alzheimers Society and SANE for people with schizophrenia whose help advocates should seek in connection with particular issues.

7   The Citizens Advice Bureaux (CABx) and the Councils of Social Service have social policy officers working on a national scale (meaning for Scotland and for the UK) to bring together and publish evidence about unmet needs and to focus public attention on problems that call for action. Some local CABx also have specialist staff providing advice and advocacy for users of the NHS. It may be useful to seek their help.

These strategies should remind advocates that they are not entirely alone in contending with public authorities. If they play an active part in their community's social and political life they will find friends and supporters. They will also meet some members of the public service professions who welcome pressures on their bosses and political masters that may enable them to provide better services.

8   If all these approaches fail, the issue may be serious enough for advocates to seek the help of politicians, first at local level, then at national levels. One of the cases discussed in Chapter Three of this book was a successful example of that kind. Advocates may also want to seek help from journalists and broadcasters.

Although these are perfectly proper things to do in a democracy, senior officials of the 'welfare state' may resent outsiders who pursue such strategies. So, before resorting to 'nuclear options' of this sort, advocates should consult their colleagues and line managers whose work may be complicated or set back by action of this kind.

Managers and their boards or managing committees should discuss these problems and work out, with their staff, the best strategies for dealing with roadblocks of this kind. They will be aware that most of these strategies are quite expensive for their agency because they make heavy demands on the time of advocates. So they will seek to work out some priorities. 'Test cases' of the kind that may affect many other people if they can be won will rank high in these priorities.

Before leaving this topic, we describe the work of GAIN, the Gateshead Advice and Information Network. It provides a hopeful conclusion to this discussion.

GAIN (Gateshead Advice and Information Network): a postscript

I met with leading spirits in this network on two occasions and am grateful for the help they gave me. They have also commented on this report on their work, but any errors it may still contain are my responsibility.

It is important to recognise that Gateshead is *different*. Things that work here may not work elsewhere. This is the deprived and battered south side of the Tyne, playing Salford to Newcastle's Manchester. From one's first glimpse of the river, marvellously cleaned up and renewed, with a great concert hall, art gallery and lifting bridge – all created mainly or wholly by Gateshead – it is clear that civic leadership thrives here. Heading across town by taxi and then walking to GAIN's offices, my taxi driver and two complete strangers on the street told me their (movingly interesting) life stories before I could get to my destination. Comradely citizenship also thrives here. And I was assured by the local advocates that their mental health services are pretty good too – better than in most neighbouring towns.

But this is England, where advocacy is frequently called for in official reports and policy statements, coming mainly from the Department of Health: *Valuing people*; *Valuing people now* (its successor); *A sure start to later life*; and *Making experiences count* are recent examples. But there is still no properly funded statutory right to it. The agencies providing it have to compete with each other, applying to many public and charitable bodies for short-term funding. On Tyneside, the collapse of Northern Rock, whose Foundation was a generous backer of local projects, makes things harder still for them.

GAIN was set up by several agencies, now seven, working, respectively, for: people with dementia; people with physical disabilities; people with visual impairments; older people (aged 50 or more); mental health service users; people with 'sensory loss'; and people with learning disabilities. Most of these were represented at my main meeting with them.

Requests for advocacy often come directly from the clients, but for people with dementia more often from public services. These agencies make considerable use of volunteer advocates. They are aware that there are other groups needing advocacy who have not yet been provided for – carers are a current concern. GAIN can help them to set up an agency of their own, but cannot do that for them. Thus their member agencies began, and largely remain, strongly rooted among the users of public services, and their parents and carers – the people who originally set them up.

Member agencies get from GAIN: information, advice, regular meetings to share experience and plan activities, a two-way link to communicate with public authorities and opportunities for coordinating their applications for funds. They have set up an Advocacy Support Network, and produced a Code of Conduct for advocacy, which helps to establish their credibility with other services. When GAIN itself was threatened with funding cuts its member agencies rallied successfully to defend it. They say they are "working towards a Gateshead where: every citizen who needs one has access to an independent advocate", and where "Advocacy services are recognised as key stakeholders in service development". Those are very ambitious aspirations.

Although under pressure from commissioners of their work to amalgamate some day and create a large 'generic' agency doing every kind of advocacy (which would be tidier and easier for bureaucrats to deal with) they are unanimous in wanting to maintain their independent specialisms, despite their precariously small sizes. "To gain respect from psychiatrists you have to show you really know something about mental illness – you're not just an all-purpose advocate." "To get someone a wheelchair that will work in their home you need to know exactly what the dimensions of each type are." They don't want to "become like a business or a social enterprise". These were the kinds of points they made. To meet their clients' needs they of course have to venture into fields outside their particular specialism, but if the problem becomes too complex they seek the help of colleagues in one of the other agencies. They see GAIN as a resource that enables them to get expert help while maintaining their independence.

I asked about their achievements as campaigners – their answer to the question posed in this chapter. Some felt their agencies, working individually, had improved things a bit. Getting ward rounds and outpatient departments in hospitals humanised and getting better food for patients were examples quoted. But Caroline Airs, Coordinator of GAIN itself, laid more emphasis on action they had taken to prevent things going wrong, rather than to put things right. By setting up repeated consultations with user groups they had got the application procedures for individual payments for social care greatly improved. (Gateshead was a pilot authority for the introduction of individual budgeting, so advocates and their clients knew a lot about it.) Caroline sits on partnership boards and other bodies that coordinate the work of Health and Social Services. There she can bring problems coming up in the work of advocates to the attention of senior managers and she occasionally gets them to come to meetings of GAIN's Advocacy Network. The danger they have to guard against is that by doing this kind of thing well they may lead public authorities to assume they do not have to consult service users and the wider community as well – only the advocacy agencies.

Other bases for collective action in Gateshead include a Mental Health Service Users' Forum, which brings users of the services together and has set up a day centre and other projects. Collective advocacy could become an important part of its job.

The local CAB – like most in this region – does not get into advocacy – "advocacy calls for a different cast of mind", I was told. The only exceptions in this region seem to be CABx in Middlesbrough and Hartlepool, which do more advocacy work.

It was suggested that, for places that lack anything equivalent to GAIN, a regional version, bringing advocacy agencies together and supporting their work in similar ways, would offer the best strategy. The Scottish Independent Advocacy Alliance aims to provide something like that for Scotland as a whole, but this may be too large a 'region' for them to exert much influence on local issues.

We are not suggesting that other places can simply install copies of GAIN, which grew, organically, from the circumstances of a particular city. But its example may inspire others to work out their own ways of achieving some of the same things. We explore those possibilities further in our next chapter.

TEN

Looking ahead

Introduction

We began this book by asking where advocacy came from. We end by asking where it's going to. As Yogi Berra, baseball coach and coiner of immortal phrases, once said: "You gotta be very careful if you don't know where you're going, because you might not get there".

People who know a lot about advocacy give two different answers to this question about its future. There are those – often inspired to play a part in the project by their own experience as users of the mental health services – who hope advocacy will reach more of the people with mental disorders and do more for them. Advocates will work more actively with groups of patients as well as with individuals, they will reach out to people in need of help who are getting no services at all, and will gain greater credibility with staff of the health and social services. These people want to 'deepen' the existing service.

Meanwhile there are those – often playing leading roles in the present advocacy services – who expect them to help growing numbers of clients with a growing variety of needs. That is already happening in the more effective parts of the service. As we have shown, an advocate who has helped a confused older lady may be asked for help by her neighbour who is mentally spry but physically disabled. Meanwhile, her agency's manager may be asked by a local authority to extend advocacy to new groups of clients – work for which the council is willing to pay. Neither finds it easy to refuse. These people are prepared to 'broaden' the service.

To deepen or broaden? It is our view that we should, cautiously, do both. But that's much too simple an answer. We are more likely to get our priorities right if we start by recalling where the service came from and consider how it meshes with other strategies for achieving some of the same things. That may enable us to clarify longer-term aims. But aims cannot be derived from facts alone. They have to be rooted in moral foundations of some sort and a vision of the society we are trying to create. Some readers will reject the vision we offer and the policies it would call for. We hope we may provoke and inspire them to formulate a vision of their own that they find more convincing.

The rise of the public service professions

In Chapter One, I told how news of Labour's landslide victory in the 1945 election reached sailors in the navy. A few weeks later we docked briefly in Portsmouth before setting off again for the Pacific war. With a 48-hour pass in my pocket, I was soon standing in the corridor of a train, packed with servicemen and stuck at Reading station. Two men wearing bowler hats and carrying brief cases hurried across the platform, hoping to get aboard. Seeing there was no hope of squeezing in, they turned away, saying, "Let's see if we can get into a first class carriage". The sailor next to me leant out of the window and bawled "First class? First class? There'll be no more bloody classes when this war's over!" – his voice echoing through the station. I sensed the support he was getting from men all along the corridor – and from unseen millions beyond. In Britain, and all over Europe, there was a pre-revolutionary frisson in the air. Governments would have to respond convincingly to the expectations of their people.

Most of our own government's promised social reforms were gradually delivered as the 'welfare state' took shape after 1948 and Britain did slowly become a more equal society in its distributions of income and wealth, in the access people had to many vital services and more generally in our social relationships. Meanwhile the growing public service professions – doctors, teachers, social workers, town planners, housing managers, social security officials and others – came to power, displacing the local gentry who had for centuries dominated our local systems of governance.

The public service professions include many hard-working, devoted and progressive people who, individually, do their best for those whom they serve. But the institutions in which they work are both products and creators of a deeply divided society.

Advocacy emerges

From the mid-1960s onwards a growing array of campaigning pressure groups developed, speaking for groups who felt excluded from the mainstream of their society – minority ethnic communities, lone parents, people with physical disabilities, gays, lesbians and others. Lay advocacy, individual and collective – in which lawyers also played a part – became a growing practice. Clearly, the people whom these advocates spoke for did not feel that the political parties or the trade unions represented them effectively. Often their demands brought them into conflict with the public services – whose staff *were* spoken for by parties and unions.

In a new environment, these campaigning groups – described rather dismissively by the political parties as 'single-issue groups' – were asserting again the hope for a fairer and more equal society, which lit up my shipmates in May 1945. Although they never got together to form a united movement, they shared the same convictions about human rights and citizenship.

People with learning disabilities and mental health difficulties came late on the advocacy scene. As they were among the most stigmatised and most excluded of all our citizens, this was not surprising. But they are gaining a growing presence in public debates about social policy and the performance of the social services; and along with that comes advocacy for individuals and for groups.

Despite the diversity of the voices competing for public attention, there was a common understanding running through their movements. They had grasped that their problems arose from their powerlessness. Investing more money, manpower and equipment in the public services would not solve these problems unless excluded people were listened to, and treated with greater respect as equal partners in any treatment or service they were to be offered. Large organisations like the police force were alleged to be 'institutionally racist' and 'sexist', both in their dealings with the public and in their treatment of their own staff. People were 'disabled', it was said, not so much by their own frailties as by buildings, employment practices and many other features of a society that discriminated against them. Lone parents were poor because society's provisions for childcare and training did not give them the help they needed.

We do not have to weigh up the justice of these claims here. The point is that they are all (with a small 'p') essentially political claims, arguing that people's handicaps are not inherent but due to the arrangements of a society that excludes them in various ways, and that these patterns should be changed. They demand a fairer, more equal society in which every citizen is treated with respect.

Recent Scottish reforms in the field of mental disorder show what can happen when powerful people listen to these demands and take them seriously. The Millan Report and the Mental Health Act that followed directly from it contain paragraph after paragraph designed to protect people with mental disorders from financial exploitation, sexual abuse, unnecessarily violent restraint, covert medication (putting medicine in their food without telling them or explaining the likely side effects), treatments, which may be damaging or terrifying imposed without consent and prolonged and unjustified incarceration.

These provisions were not the whims of starry-eyed reformers. They arose from the fact that the Millan Committee included among its members people who had long experience as users of the mental health services; and the Committee took a lot of trouble to tour Scotland and listen to users of these services and the people who care for them. They concluded that a new Mental Health Act was needed and one of its main purposes must be to protect mental health service users from the mental health services.

Free and independent advocacy for all mental health service users – whether in hospital or in the community, and whether subject to compulsion or not – was one of the rights conferred by the new Act. This was an essentially political step, intended to tackle problems arising from the powerlessness of patients.

In the health services these movements on behalf of service users have joined forces with movements among service providers who believe that 'health' is not a commodity dispensed by experts to their 'customers', but an achievement of doctors and patients working together. Julian Tudor Hart,[1] in the book briefly described in our notes on Further Reading, is one of those who have developed this argument. Peter Tyrer and Derek Steinberg,[2] also noted under Further Reading, describe cognitive-behavioural methods of treatment that have developed recently: "The hierarchy of medicine is alien to the behavioural therapist"; "a two-way contract between treaters and treated cannot develop in a hierarchical atmosphere". Serious relapse after treatment, they argue, is less common among patients who have taken greater responsibility for their treatment. David Brandon, who had been both treater and treated in the mental health services, put it this way:

> Here are two ordinary people, neither of them walking six inches above the ground ... engaging in a complex transaction about 'sickness' and treatment. One is usually in pain and suffering; the other may have relevant skills and knowledge. During that transaction they contribute different perspectives and may disagree. Neither tries to manipulate the other to win control. Instead, they move gently towards compromises and agreements. They move towards sharing information and respect for each other's position. They are humble rather than arrogant; aware of what they do not know rather than what they know. In particular, the practitioner should respect the

autonomy of the patient and learn something of his or her whole life.

Other ways of shifting the balance of power

Advocacy is only one of the ways in which the powerlessness of many users of our public services may be put right. And pretty flimsy it is. The agency that has been the source of most of the case studies and examples in this book employs only 16 staff – amounting to a full-time equivalent of about a dozen – plus quite a lot of unpaid volunteers. It serves a population of 185,000. So we should note other strategies that help to make public services more accountable to their most vulnerable users and consider the part that advocacy plays within this broader pattern.

Markets

The main response of Conservative governments to these problems – since developed further by Labour governments for England, but less vigorously in Scotland – was to create markets and 'market-like' conditions, which would compel public services to compete with each other for 'customers'. Public services were contracted out to commercial and voluntary providers. The operations of services still provided by the state were priced and the funds flowing to them tracked so that the costs and outputs of particular procedures could be compared and their productivity improved. Information about their performance was assembled and published so that their users could decide for themselves which to turn to – often with help from professional advisers. (General practitioners were to play this crucial role in the health services.) Targets, tests and indicators of many kinds were invented to motivate the providers of services, measure their progress and help their 'customers' make choices; and money, it was planned, would ultimately follow demand.

The authors of some excellent books[3] have argued that these policies have been professionally, economically and morally disastrous. The central flame fuelling their anger is a conviction that a commercial morality is inappropriate for a public service, distorts professional and political decisions, and corrupts behaviour.

It is our view that these criticisms have a lot to be said for them in the fields of health and education, and even more in the field of prison policy, but less, perhaps, in the fields of housing and residential care. By posing these complex issues as a choice between the public and the private sectors, critics of 'marketisation' oversimplify the issue. They also neglect altogether the voluntary sector, which plays so large a part in advocacy and in many other fields – including the lifeboat service and mountain rescue where everyone seems happy with this arrangement.

Those who most fiercely defend the public services from market influences presumably rely on good managers and democratically elected politicians to put things right if people depending on these services are neglected, ill treated or denied their rights. But the democratic state also has defects – particularly for the poorest and most vulnerable people, and for ethnic and other minorities not popular with 'middle England' and its tabloid press. (Cases described in this book provide too many examples of that.) The inverse care laws operating in many services are a scandal that has to be addressed. It is not good enough just to dig in and defend every feature of 'Nye Bevan's NHS' and its counterparts in other services. (Bevan himself would not have done so.) If western parliamentary democracy was a sufficient guarantee of social justice, voluntary groups advocating for people excluded in various ways from society's mainstream would not have been steadily growing since the Child Poverty Action Group and Shelter set the pattern more than 40 years ago. So what other strategies can protect the most vulnerable people?

Direct payments and individual budgets for social care services

This is a growing practice that local authorities are being encouraged to adopt. It is another kind of 'marketisation', but with the crucial difference that the state can target buying power to the people whose needs seem to be greatest. Service users' needs and resources are assessed, and they are allocated funds which enable them to choose their own providers of services and make their own arrangements with them. Our experience suggests this can work very well for people with physical disabilities who have the support of strong and loyal families. But, where service users have other severe difficulties and no close friends or relatives to help them, they will need expert, friendly, *long-term* advice and support; something more than the services of an advocate whose job is to help people with particular problems and get on to the next case.

Strategies for empowering service users

These may range from 'community-*based* services' giving their users strong representation on governing bodies where they help to select staff, secure funds and decide policies, to 'community *ownership*' giving users complete control of an agency or large parts of it. Some housing associations work in this cooperative fashion. The Edinburgh Users Forum, which we described earlier in this book, is run very effectively by current and former users of the mental health services with help from a small 'civil service' of professional supporters.

The state can find, inspire and support communities and groups that are prepared to take on these responsibilities. But such projects will always be patchy – the state cannot 'roll out' a nationwide programme of this kind. Meanwhile, 'community' includes everyone in the area or the group concerned, including the mafia if they operate there – drug dealers and illicit money lenders. So audit and regulation, in which elected councillors play some part, will be required to ensure there are procedures that help to keep people honest, efficient and accountable – just as are needed for state services that may also fall into the wrong hands.

'Community' has no inherent virtue. It can be a powerful excluder of minorities. The old people's club that runs a publicly funded community hall too often excludes young people from the premises – or even the old people in the next street or tower block. Again, effective supervision by people reporting to a broader electorate will be needed to control these tendencies.

Public service professions can take special steps to help those who use their services

This is an important but too rare contribution that the professions can make. Planning Aid is a charity staffed by volunteers from the town planning profession. They are prepared not to represent but to advise people – helping them to cope with the planning system they operate during their working week. Lawyers may do 'pro bono' work without charge for needy clients and some of them work in law centres that employ solicitors specialising in different fields, including mental health – mainly serving people who are entitled to legal aid. Other public service professions should consider whether they could work in the same ways.

Human rights law

The Human Rights Act has brought European human rights law to Britain. Some have argued that its scope should be greatly extended to confer many economic and social rights.[4] This may seem a ponderous and slow-moving machine for the ordinary citizen to mobilise. But a brave prisoner, supported by a few expert witnesses, used the Act to bring slopping out to an end in jails throughout Britain. With good legal advice, this will sometimes be another means to social justice. It has the advantage that it can be brought to bear on test cases that eventually confer new rights on people throughout the country, not only on the individuals who sought the help of the courts.

User surveys

If you take your car to a big repair shop you are liable to receive a phone call soon after, asking you how you would rate the service provided by its telephonist, its receptionist, its mechanics and the lady who prepared your bill. Was the waiting room comfortable? The coffee drinkable? Would you take your car there again? Buy another from them? Recommend a friend to do likewise? But if you take your own body to the nearest big hospital – a *teaching* hospital – does anyone ask you if the experience made you feel better or worse? Did the doctors explain what they were doing, and why? Could you understand what they said? Was the food eatable? The ward clean? Did anyone bring a bedpan or give you a wash when you needed it? The state has a good deal to learn from some of the better practice in the private sector.

Community care

Most important in the longer run is the hope that we may develop what might be called *real community care*. Community care has too often been interpreted as professional services provided for people living in their own homes. But there are communities in which people provide a lot of care and support for neighbours who fall ill, injure themselves or experience lifelong disabilities. Such neighbourly care is not a substitute for public service; indeed, it thrives best where public services are good. People are more likely to help a neighbour who is going through a mental breakdown if they know there are good health services ready to take over if they get out of their depth.

On a small island where I spend a lot of time (permanent residents numbering about 70) people noticed when a neighbour fell into depression; got him on his feet and cleaned his house up for him; eventually got him to hospital and visited him regularly; fed his dog and took it for walks; then supported him when he came home. A child who had Down's syndrome played very happily with the other children who took good care of him. When they set off on the ferry each morning to start at the local primary school the parents of this boy approached the headmistress and said he wanted to come to her school with his friends. "He can't talk. But in the family we use a sign language for the deaf which we all understand." "That's fine", replied the head. "I and my colleagues will learn his signs – and so will all the children in this school." And they did and very popular the boy became. The head was saying, in effect, that a boy with this disability was an asset to her school. All her children should learn that people have widely varying abilities, but all have a contribution to make to their community.

While this island may inspire us, what we need is a whole country that is more accepting of deviance, and kinder towards those who experience such difficulties and disorders. In the bigger cities and the impersonal suburbs that house most of our people, that kind of support is most likely to grow up around groups concerned with a particular illness or disability. We should remember that 60% of NHS spending is devoted to long-term conditions – not hip replacements and injuries but diabetes and dementia. That means there are lots of people out there who probably know better than most doctors how to manage these conditions and can certainly give new patients more time than the doctors. By finding and fostering these groups and putting people in touch with them patients can get good advice, continuing support and advocacy when they need it.

These are not the only strategies that can help to empower and support people who may feel lonely and helpless. Childline is a telephone service that receives thousands of calls every year from children who are bullied, children who have difficulties with their parents and children who are abused in various ways. The service provides valuable advice and support. Other helplines do likewise.

Less attractive is the growing practice of litigation against the health service and the schools by people seeking compensation for the mistakes they make – taking millions of pounds out of the funds that could otherwise be devoted to improving patient care and teaching. Too often, people who feel injured can find no one who will listen to them. Public service staff have probably been ordered to say nothing – and on no account to apologise, which may be all that people are asking for. So aggrieved service users may feel that this individualistic, 'customer-style' strategy is the only one open to them.

Advocates should be alert to the many other methods and resources available to help their clients. They should put their clients in touch with them when that is helpful and particularly support the development of constructive, community-building strategies that ultimately help all of us.

Looking ahead

What conclusions can we come to about the future of advocacy?

We should start modestly, recognising that there are many other procedures and movements that may help to gain a hearing for our clients. Like advocacy, these strategies can help the public service professions to do a better job and gain for themselves stronger roots in the communities they serve. That way, their patients, clients, tenants and pupils may march alongside them when the next assault is made on them. We should put our own clients in touch with these movements and strategies when it seems helpful to do so – and particularly with those that appeal to people as citizens and enable them to improve the services on which all of us may ultimately depend. If advocacy only provides a megaphone to enable the sharper 'customers' to get their mothers into the *best* care homes, their daughters into the *best* secondary schools, it will not be a cause worth devoting one's life to.

The Millan Committee recommended – and the Scottish Parliament followed its advice – that, to be genuinely independent, advocacy must be securely funded by the state and provided by agencies that do nothing else. It is surprising how many people elsewhere have written and spoken learnedly about the need for advocacy without confronting this simple fact.

There are many people in the public service professions who want to give those who depend on them a voice that will be listened to. Advocates should look out for these people and work closely with them.

It is possible to do a useful job of advocacy as a nurse or a social worker, or as a member of a precariously funded voluntary agency that pays the rent by earning money for other services it provides. No one should discourage anyone from acting as an advocate. But each has their limits. Nurses and social workers have to decide to which patient or client they should give priority – and that may not be the one who most needs the help of an advocate. They have to maintain good relations with colleagues without whose help they cannot do their own jobs effectively. Small voluntary agencies cannot displease the public authorities that pay for their work unless they are prepared to go out of business over a point of principle. So there will be times when all these people need to pass the ball to an independent advocate who does not have to worry about such things. Several of the cases we have described show how grateful other professionals sometimes are when they can bring in an advocate who negotiates for them with other beasts in the bureaucratic jungle on behalf of people they are trying to help. Much of advocacy is 'brokerage' that helps the big bureaucracies of the 'welfare state' to work more constructively together.

To give whole-hearted commitment to their client's cause, advocates have to bear in mind that the ultimate responsibility for any decisions to be made will always remain with the professionals. It is not for advocates to decide what would be in their clients' best interest, or which user of public services deserves priority over the rest. They are not bidding to take over the professionals' power. They believe that the professionals will make better decisions if they really understand how their patients or clients feel and what they really want.

Advocates help their clients to gain greater respect and acceptance, both from the authorities they depend on – their doctors, social workers, parents, employers, etc – and from the community at large whose support and kindness is, in the long run, most important of all. The authorities will respond better when the community insists that they do so. So public education is a continuing part of the job of advocates, their managers and board members. That will call for active participation in local community groups and a willingness to run courses, to speak in public, give interviews for the local press and radio, and much else.

Most of an advocate's work will probably be done for individual clients. But they should not be content with reinforcing the demands of individual 'customers'. They want also to help to change and improve the services and systems on which we may all some day have to depend. That means building a collective sense of citizenship, which comes through working with volunteers, helping groups of people who have experience of the services concerned and – once again – getting out into the community.

There are many different kinds of independent advocacy – citizen advocacy, peer advocacy, group advocacy and so on. Advocates of the kind described in this book should welcome them all, for each has an important contribution to make. None of them should be tempted to claim the moral high ground. Likewise there are professions the advocate encounters whose members regard themselves as advocates for their clients and patients. We should all welcome that. The more people there are who respect and support those who depend on their services, the better pleased we should be.

Hector Mackenzie's challenge to all public services – recorded in Chapter Two of this book – to provide independent advocacy for those who depend on them has not gone away. The more effective advocacy services are already extending the range of clients for whom they act and therefore also the range of agencies they have to deal with. They are 'broadening' their service. That will eventually pose questions about the kind of agency that would provide the most effective base on which to build an expanding advocacy service. An agency that has made its reputation by working for frail and stigmatised groups of people may not be the best one to choose. We should therefore consider what others might be available. Some of our Citizens Advice Bureaux might fill the bill. But others would not. Advice and advocacy call for different casts of mind, as we were told in Gateshead.

I believe that the Millan Committee got it right when it discussed how to launch this service. After long debate it decided that advocacy should be provided, not by the state, the private sector or some nationwide voluntary body, but by local voluntary agencies that were already doing this kind of work. The agency from which our own sprang served people who had Alzheimer's disease. Others began from a concern for people with schizophrenia, learning disabilities or other conditions. These agencies have developed in varied ways that reflect their own particular strengths and the needs they encounter in their territory. As the value of advocacy comes to be more widely recognised, we should look first for groups with particular loyalties and expertise who can be helped to provide their own advocacy service for people they probably know better than anyone else. A fully independent, generic service, doing nothing but advocacy, may come later. But we should not be trying to build an advocacy empire. Service personnel and ex-service personnel – of whom there are many in the area we know best – have higher rates of mental health difficulties than most people. The radio every morning tells us why that might be so. Rather than trying to extend their own services directly to them, advocates should start by talking with the charities helping service personnel and their families, and see if there is any help that experienced advocates could offer that would strengthen the support they are already giving to these families.

Whether considering future paths that advocacy may take or looking to other strategies for achieving some of the same things, we should choose those that are most likely to strengthen our roles as citizens with collective responsibilities, not just customers fighting our own corner and thereby excluding other less aggressive or less fortunate people. Advocacy should not become part of the systems that divide a society and disempower its more vulnerable citizens. It should help to reverse, not reinforce, the inverse care laws that so often operate within our public services. The concerns for human rights and social justice that inspired the pioneers in this field must not be forgotten.

Notes

[1] Julian Tudor Hart, *The political economy of health care*, Bristol, The Policy Press, 2006, p 9.

[2] Peter Tyrer and Derek Steinberg, *Models for mental disorder* (4th edn), Chichester, John Wiley, 2005, pp 91-2 and 95.

[3] For example, Julian Tudor Hart, *The political economy of health care*, Bristol, The Policy Press, 2006; Alysson Pollock, *NHS plc: The privatisation of our health care*, London, Verso, 2004; Vivien Stern, *Creating criminals: Prisons and people in a market society*, London, Zed Books, 2006; Stuart Weir, *Unequal Britain: Human rights as a route to social justice,* London, Politico's, 2006.

[4] Stuart Weir, *Unequal Britain: Human rights as a route to social justice*, London, Politico's, 2006.

Further reading

We conclude with some suggestions for further reading about the main themes of this book.

On the health services and community care

Robin Means, Sally Richards and Randall Smith, *Community care: Policy and practice* (4th edn), Basingstoke, Palgrave Macmillan, 2008.
An up-to-date textbook on community care in England for adults with many different needs. Little is said about advocacy, but many of the issues touched on in our book are dealt with: empowerment of service users, human rights law, direct payments and individual budgets, the 'marketisation' of public services and so on.

John Welshman and Jan Walmsley (eds), *Community care in perspective: Care, control and citizenship*, Basingstoke, Palgrave Macmillan, 2006.
A dozen authors trace the development of care outside residential institutions from 1948 to 2001, mainly in England, but with useful chapters on other countries – particularly the US. Essentially a history of ideas and the social movements that carried our thinking forward. References to advocacy deal mainly with service user groups, parent groups and citizen advocacy. None describes the Scottish version.

Julian Tudor Hart, *The political economy of health care*, Bristol, The Policy Press, 2006.
A marvellous account of the NHS from the perspective of lifelong work as a general practitioner in a working-class community. Mixes extensive scientific knowledge with innovative, community-based clinical thinking and a passionate defence of the original values of the National Health Service.

Scottish Executive, *Building a health service fit for the future*, May 2005.
Explains the Scottish government's plans for the development of health services, posing questions and presenting principles that are important in any developed country.

Howard Stoate, MP and Bryan Jones, *Challenging the citadel: Breaking the hospitals' grip on the NHS*, London, Fabian Society, 2007.
An interesting pamphlet that makes an important contribution to current debates about the future of the NHS.

Allyson M. Pollock, *NHS plc: The privatisation of our health care*, London, Verso, 2004.

A polemical but well researched attack on the privatisation and 'marketisation' of the NHS and their destructive effects. But without any recognition that other means for making the public service professions accountable must be found if market solutions are to be resisted.

On mental health and learning disabilities: Scottish law and policy

The Millan Report: *New directions: Report on the Review of the Mental Health (Scotland) Act, 1984*, Scottish Executive, 2001 – with a good website.

The progressive report that led to the development of the Scottish service described in this book. Bruce Millan's Committee had to focus mainly on legal powers and procedures. Their well-written report combines humanity with tough realism.

Hilary Patrick, *Mental health, incapacity and the law in Scotland,* Haywards Heath and Edinburgh, Tottel Publishing, 2006.

Not a book to read through – or to buy (too expensive) – but this is the essential, massive work of reference on the subjects of its title; clearly and beautifully written by a lawyer who played a key part in the work of the Millan Committee.

On mental health and learning disabilities: policy and practice

Peter Tyrer and Derek Steinberg, *Models for mental disorder: Conceptual models in psychiatry* (4th edn), Chichester, John Wiley, 2005.

Psychiatrists think about mental disorders in quite different ways, bring different theories to bear and use different strategies for treating the same symptoms. This book describes and distinguishes the disorder, the psychodynamic, the cognitive-behavioural and the social models, playing fair by each. Brilliant final chapter on the ways in which these strategies may be brought most fruitfully together. Clearly and wittily written.

David Pilgrim, *Key concepts in mental health*, London, SAGE, 2005.

Gives brief, clear, humane explanations of the concepts used in this field, divided into three sections dealing with mental disorders, mental health services, and the broader social aspects and implications of the field. Good, brief reading lists for each of the 50 items covered. They do not include advocacy.

Kathleen Jones, *Experience in mental health: Community care and social policy,* London, SAGE, 1988.

This (she tells me) is the last of Kathleen Jones's many books on the history of our mental health services. It includes excellent chapters on American, Italian, Chinese and Nigerian experience, a report on a small but important study tracing what happened to people discharged from long-stay mental hospitals, critical appraisals of some of the heroes of progressive mental care and a magisterial concluding chapter on the reforms required (most of them *still* required). But no role for advocacy or the users of mental health services.

Helen Lester and John Glasby, *Mental health policy and practice,* Basingstoke, Palgrave Macmillan, 2006.

A textbook on the subjects in its title. Helpful if you like lots of 'boxed' summaries of the points being made. Few references to advocacy but a useful chapter on 'User involvement' in the mental health services.

On advocacy and related issues

Barry Gray and Robin Jackson (eds), *Advocacy and learning disability,* London, Jessica Kingsley, 2002.

Fourteen chapters by 21 authors on the history of advocacy in this field, some of them excellent. See, particularly, two by Michael Kendrick on the philosophy and politics of advocacy in this field, one by Mike Pochin who is realistically frank about the difficulties of developing citizen advocacy schemes, and one by Deborah Baillie and Veronica Strachan who describe the early days of the Scottish system.

Dorothy Atkinson, *Advocacy: A review,* Brighton, Pavilion Publishing, for Joseph Rowntree Foundation, 1999.

A good description of the main types and traditions of advocacy and their history till 1998. Good on the evaluation of advocacy and on advocacy by social workers.

David Brandon, *Innovation without change? Consumer power in psychiatric services,* Basingstoke, Macmillan Education, 1991.

A vividly written account of the development of various forms of advocacy for people with mental health and learning disabilities by a scholar who played a part in the story as a user of mental health services, practitioner, advocate and teacher. He never forgets the importance of power relationships in the mental health services.

David Brandon with Althea and Toby Brandon, *Advocacy: Power to people with disabilities*, Birmingham, Venture Press, 1995.
A later book from the Brandon family takes the story further, giving good descriptions of the different kinds of advocacy to be seen in the 1990s. Excellent final conclusions.

Rick Henderson and Mike Pochin, *A right result? Advocacy, justice and empowerment*, Bristol, The Policy Press, 2001.
Another and more up-to-date review of the development of various brands of advocacy for individuals (not groups). Written from an English viewpoint. Good on training and evaluation.

Peter Beresford and Suzy Croft, *Citizen involvement: A practical guide for change*, Basingstoke, Macmillan, 1993.
A good, practical, how-to-do-it guide for community activists, social workers and others who want to involve and empower groups of citizens. Includes a brief but useful section on advocacy.

The journal *Social Policy and Society*, vol 7, no 2 for April 2008, has a themed section with five articles on 'Choice or voice? The impact of consumerism on public services'. For readers prepared to hack their way through thickets of academic jargon these articles offer thoughtful ideas about the implications of the growth of individualised 'customer relations' between public services and the people who use them.

Joe Kenyon, *A passion for justice: The stories of Joe Kenyon*, Nottingham Trent University, Trent Editions, 2003.
The life, told in stories, of a natural advocate. Kenyon was a miner, trade unionist, teacher, welfare rights adviser and community activist who battled till the end of his life to help people he felt were being unjustly treated. All told in a gentle, compelling Barnsley accent.

Action for Advocacy, an organisation speaking for agencies doing advocacy work, produces a quarterly magazine, Planet Advocacy (£15 a year), which provides a good, easy-to-read English perspective on independent advocacy. For more information, consult www.actionforadvocacy.org.uk

Index

Supplementary Benefits Commission,
13
Sweden, 22

T

Terminology and language, 38–39, 94
Thatcher, Margaret, 15
Trade Unions, 13–16, 135, 146–47
Trades Union Congress, 13
Tressell, Robert, 9
Tudor Hart, Julian, 10, 12, 85, 148
Tyrer, Peter, 148

U

United States of America (US), 20, 22,
125

W

Webb, Beatrice, 8–9, 11,17
Webb, Sidney, 9, 11, 17
Winnicott, Donald, 20
Woolfson, Peter, viii